WEIGHT WA

New Complete Personalpoint Cookbook

#2024

WW Simple, Quick And Tasty Smart Points Meals For Everyone Who Wants To Lose Weight And Live A Healthy Life

By Jenesis Katrine

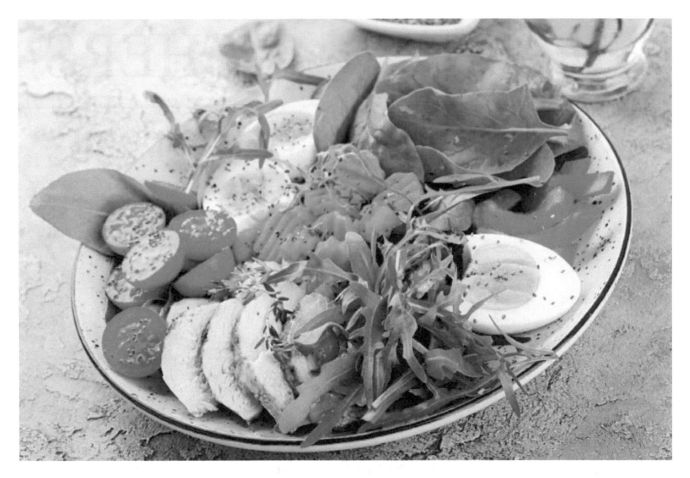

NEW COMPLETE COOKBOOK 2024

Copyright © Jenesis Katrine

Table of Contents

Introduction

Weight Watchers is unquestionably the most widely used weight loss program on the planet. Weight Watchers has built its strategy on a strong basis of weight loss research for over 45 years. The New Weight Watchers Diet Cookbook offers you over 600 delicious and nutritious recipes to help you stay on track with the PointsPlusTM program, Weight Watchers' newest and most scientifically supported weight control program. Below is a summary of Weight Watchers' approach to exercise, behavior change, and weight loss (including the PointsPlusTM program) to help you make choices that will improve your health and increase your chances of success.

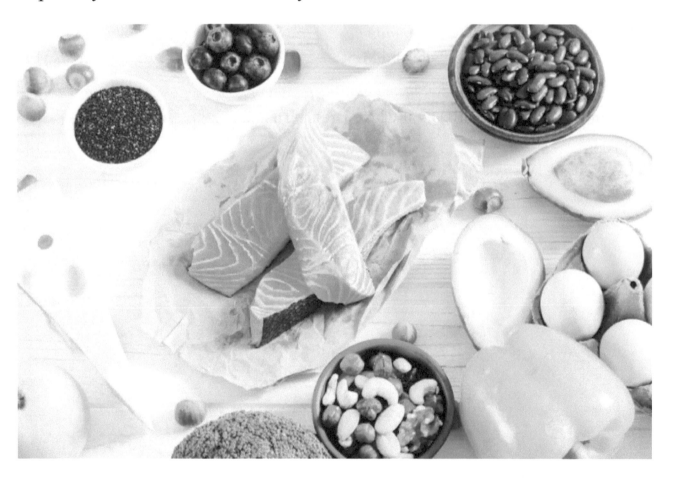

What is Weight Watchers?

If you've never heard of Weight Watchers, it's a program that encourages individuals to live better lifestyles and has Oprah's support. The program offers numerous additional advantages despite the fact that the majority of participants join in order to reduce their weight. It encourages healthy practices like drinking water, working out, meditating, and getting enough sleep. According to U.S. News & World Report, this diet program ranks first in the area of best diet program, second in the category of best weight-loss diet, and third in the category of easiest diets to follow.

By adjusting a person's daily calorie intake to their unique demographic traits, Weight Watchers encourages secure and efficient weight reduction (age, weight, height, and gender). Every eaten item has a certain number of points. The good point value of proteins is lower than that of carbohydrates and saturated fats. If an item is on a list of foods with 0 points, you are free to consume as much as you want of it. You should experience weight reduction if you adhere to your daily point allocation (or less). The goal is to strengthen your ability to make decisions and, with practice, make better decisions instinctively.

How does Weight Watchers Work?

You may lose weight with the help of the excellent weight-loss program Weight Watchers in a healthy and effective manner. However, some diet regimens focus on limiting your calorie intake and advising you on what you can and cannot eat. While this could be effective for some people, it might be difficult for them to avoid their favorite foods constantly. Furthermore, buying food may be difficult while following a certain diet plan. Weight Watchers will function differently. It recognizes that you have a lot going on in your life and can't afford to sit around and look for expensive things or difficult-to-find ingredients to be healthy. This one is based on Smart Points, which let you choose the meals that are most beneficial to you and encourage healthy eating while avoiding unhealthy food. Being aware of your particular eating patterns is key to following this diet. You will be given a certain amount of points to utilize each day, and you may choose how you use them. You may even develop your own recipes and calculate the point values, and each meal you choose will be assigned a different point value. If you actually want to cheat throughout the week or can't resist a big celebration, this routine enables you to. You'll learn that you can still eat them and still count them toward your daily point totals. If you use these little shortcuts wisely the rest of the day, your hard work won't be undone. Weight Watchers includes more than just planning out the wholesome foods you should consume during the week. These include of going to meetings and adding more exercise to your daily routine. Weight Watchers meetings are a unique aspect that has helped the organization succeed in various ways. The goal of these sessions is to make you accountable for the weight you have set out to lose. These are often conducted once a week and provide you the chance to meet others in your area who share your interests. You may enter and get a confidential weight assessment before meeting with others to exchange information and find motivation to go on. Your level of activity will be crucial when following the Weight Watchers program. Even if this has changed a little since the program's beginning, it is still essential to go out there and partake in a variety of activities to keep your body healthy and enable you to lose as much weight as you can. The wonderful thing about Weight Watchers is that you can use it to completely change your way of life. This tool does not need you to put in a lot of effort to complete tasks that are impossible in order to get the desired results. To get the desired results, Weight Watchers urges you to adopt a new lifestyle that includes eating the appropriate meals, exercising regularly, and acquiring the proper information.

Why Choose Weight Watchers?

You may choose from a variety of really successful diet strategies. Some people would advise you to cut down on carbohydrates, while others will advise you to cut back on fat. Some are good for your health, while others are hard on your body and difficult to maintain. Because it provides specialized solutions, Weight Watchers distinguishes itself from comparable programs.

For the reasons listed below, you should choose Weight Watchers as your weight-loss program:

Lose a few more pounds. Others who adhere to a program like Weight Watchers often have more success with weight loss than people who opt for different strategies.

This is so because it is simple to carry out and because weekly meetings provide participants with support and direction.

Flexibility On Weight Watchers, there is a lot of flexibility. You have complete control over what, when, and how much food you consume based on the points you have available. You have a lot of control over your fitness routine, how often you get together, and whether those encounters take place in person or online. It is instantly clear what the optimum course of action for this tactic is.

Weight Watchers is more than simply a diet program. It all comes down to changing one's behaviors in order to lose weight gradually and healthily. You'll learn which foods lead to weight gain and health problems and how to replace them with better options. Your perspective on exercise will change as you learn to like it and incorporate it into your daily routine. Your current problems with stress and sleep will get priority attention.

On this diet, you are allowed to eat anything you want, so feel free to sometimes treat yourself to some of your favorite comfort foods. However, you must make better decisions when it comes to

On a diet with a limited number of points, you may still enjoy some of your favorite meals.

Making it a part of your regular routine You might simply include this eating regimen into your daily routine. You have access to scrumptious, filling real food. You might opt to work out every day or do routine tasks like cleaning instead of spending hours each day at the gym. You are allowed to eat whatever you choose in moderation as long as it doesn't go above the meal limitations.

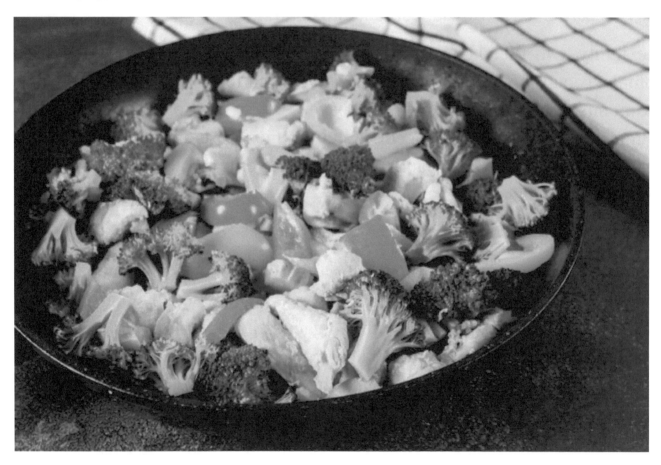

You are allowed to dine at restaurants while on this plan. On this diet, eating out sometimes is OK, but doing so consistently is not. It recognizes that there will be occasions when you go out with friends and family and that you will be OK without destroying all your hard work as long as you make the proper decisions for the rest of the day and don't overeat at the restaurant.

Attending weekly meetings will help you maintain focus on your strategy and perhaps meet individuals who can assist you along the way. When things become rough, the people you encounter along the journey may provide encouragement and support. On any of your prior eating regimens, it was challenging to maintain this level of enthusiasm.

Only Weight Watchers provides its members with as much variety and assistance in their weight reduction journey as it does. Whether you've attempted to lose weight in the past without much success and are now prepared to give it another go, see if Weight Watchers can assist you.

The Smart Points

In 2016, Weight Watchers implemented a number of changes to its points system. Their software has been criticized for placing too much emphasis on users' point totals and not enough on the healthiness of the food they were eating.

Following the Weight Watchers guidelines might make it difficult for people to get enough of certain nutrients or prevent them from opting for meals that are lower in healthy fats and proteins. For this reason, Weight Watchers launched its "Smart Points" and "Beyond the Scale" initiatives in 2016.

Since Smart Points simplify point calculation, you'll be more likely to choose for healthier options. You may improve your mood, decrease your weight, and boost your energy all at once by doing this. Higher point values have been assigned to formerly lower-scoring foods, such as those rich in sugar and saturated fat. Scores may be lowered by eating fresh veggies and lean proteins.

Though you'll still have free reign over what goes into your body, keeping track of points will encourage you to prioritize nutritious options at mealtimes.

Reduce your consumption of sugar and saturated fat and increase your protein intake, and you'll get more points under the new system.

Weight Watchers' Activity Points have been renamed "FitPoints," and they will now be awarded in proportion to the amount of exercise you get each week. Scheduled exercises and mundane housekeeping might both be on the agenda for the day.

When you join Weight Watchers, you'll get 49 bonus points to use anyway you choose, on top of your regular point total. This is perfect for your cheat day or for those times when you just can't hold in your hunger. These extra calories will still be included towards Smart Points, but to varying degrees depending on the person. Age, gender, weight-loss motivation, and activity levels are all factors that might be considered.

How do Weight Watchers points work?

To lose weight with Weight Watchers, you will focus on making healthier meal choices rather than cutting out whole food groups. This eating plan understands that you'll have cravings for sweets on occasion and that telling you to avoid them would just make things worse. So long as they are part of a well-balanced diet, these foods are allowed on the Weight Watchers plan. You will be given a point system to use when you join Weight Watchers. You may use your current weight and desired amount of use in the method to inform your decision-making. To encourage healthier eating habits, you have this many points to spend each day. The goal is to limit daily point intake, and each meal will be assigned a point value.

You can have some of the sweets, but if you're getting close to the end of the day and only have five points left, it would be wise to choose an apple instead of the piece of cake that would put you over your point goal because of its higher value (15 points). You decide how to spend the points, and there are guides to assist you determine how many points are associated with different food choices. You may plan ahead of time to pick clean and healthful products that will keep you inside your points limit without compromising nutrition if you want a piece of cake throughout the day (perhaps you are going to a birthday party). You need to be very careful around here. Extreme calorie restriction is an approach used by some too passionate dieters. People often think that if they cut their calorie intake in half, they would see rapid results in their weight loss efforts. The issue here, though, is that cutting calories also means cutting out on healthy food for the body. To avoid any mishaps, you need to use extraordinary care. Your daily point totals will be lower on days when you aren't as hungry or too busy to eat as much as you should. You don't have to force yourself to eat anymore. But you should aim to go close to your daily point totals so that your body gets adequate fuel. These factors will be critical in determining which items you can eat while on this diet. You will be focusing on the points you earn rather than the calories you ingest. It's based on the macro and micronutrients in the meals you plan to eat. Fewer points are assigned to a food item if it is rich in good macro and microelements like protein, acceptable carbs, and healthy vitamins. To put it another way, you may have more of it spread out throughout the course of the day. However, you will be able to use more points for purchases that are heavy in calories, carbs, and saturated fats. In general, you'll be encouraged to make better food choices and discouraged from eating certain types of food, while yet being given the freedom to enjoy some less-than-healthy foods on a limited basis. Following these guidelines may help you choose the healthiest options when it comes to what you put in your body. You can still indulge in sweets every once in a while, but you'll find that the healthier options are more satisfying overall. This is because you'll be able to consume more of them without exceeding your point total.

The Advantages of Smart Points

Smart Points are one of the main reasons why the Weight Watchers program is so successful in helping people lose weight.

The following are some of the most compelling arguments in favor of using this system:

- Smart Points are a helpful tool for making nutritious meal choices. If you choose foods that are heavy in sugars and saturated fats, you will be punished, while those who go for the healthier options will not.
- The Smart Points program debunked the dangerous belief that increased physical activity justifies one's increased caloric intake. Many individuals exaggerate how much effort they put into maintaining a healthy weight, making it difficult for them to cut calories when they eat poorly. If you want to lose weight with Smart Points, you'll have to keep your physical activity and food intake distinct.
- The emphasis of these Smart Points will be on making healthy choices. Although losing weight is important, you will learn that maintaining your ideal weight is more about adopting a healthy lifestyle overall than it is about obsessive calorie tracking and food preoccupation.

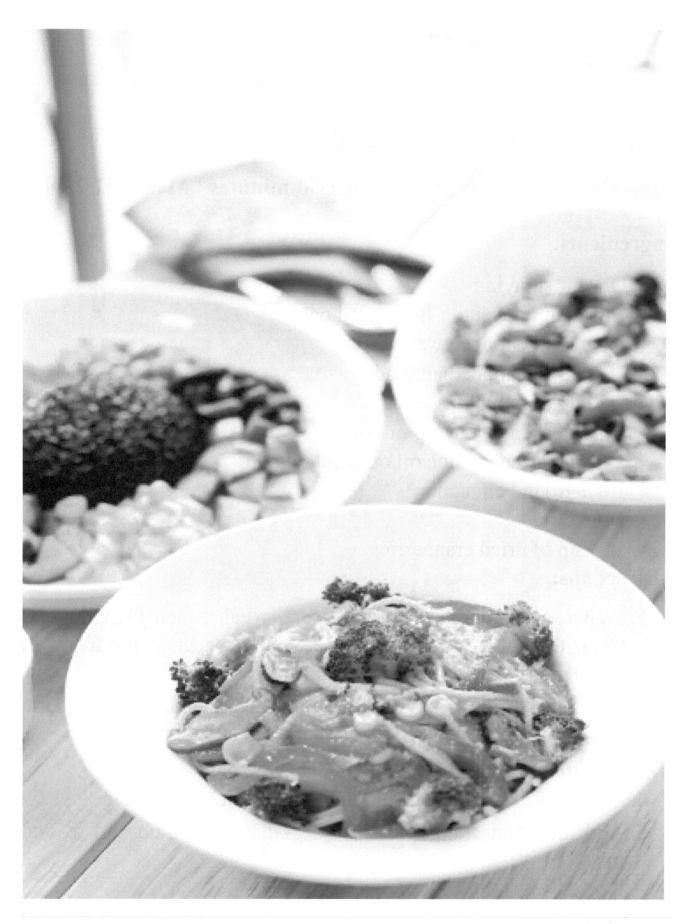

Breakfasts

Gluten-Free Granola Cereal

Prep time: 7 minutes | Cook time: 30 minutes | Makes 31/2 cups of

Ingredients:

- Oil, for spraying
- 1-1/2 cups of gluten-free rolled oats
- 1/2 cup of chopped walnuts
- 1/2 cup of chopped almonds
- 1/2 cup of pumpkin seeds
- 1/4 cup of maple syrup or honey
- 1 tbsp toasted sesame oil or vegetable oil
- 1 tsp ground cinnamon
- 1/2 tsp salt
- 1/2 cup of dried cranberries

Directions:

1. Prepare a temperature of 250 degrees Fahrenheit (121 degrees C) in the air fryer. Put some parchment paper in the air fryer basket and spray some cooking spray on it.
2. Combine the oats, nuts, seeds, oil, spices, and salt in a large Cup. Mix in the maple syrup, sesame oil, and cinnamon.
3. Distribute the ingredients evenly in the basket.
4. Stir every 10 minutes for the first 30 minutes of cooking.
5. Add the dried cranberries to the granola in a Cup and toss to mix.

6. Put in an airtight container when they have cooled to room temperature.

Per Serving

Calories: 322 | fat: 17g | protein: 11g | carbs: 35g | fiber: 6g | sodium: 170mg

Butternut Squash and Ricotta Frittata

Prep time: 10 minutes | Cook time: 33 minutes | Serves 2 to 3
Ingredients:

- 1 cup of cubed (1/2-inch) butternut squash (51/2 OZs / 156 g)
- 2 tbsp olive oil
- Kosher salt and freshly ground black pepper, to taste
- 4 fresh sage leaves, thinly sliced
- 6 large eggs, lightly beaten
- 1/2 cup of ricotta cheese
- Cayenne pepper

Directions:

1. Salt and black pepper the squash, then put it in a dish with the olive oil and toss again to coat everything evenly. Place the squash in a cake pan and sprinkle the sage over the squash. Throw the dish into the air fryer and cook it for 10 minutes at 400 degrees Fahrenheit (204 degrees Celsius). After adding the sage, give everything a good stir and continue cooking for another 3 minutes, or until the squash is soft and beginning to caramelize around the edges.

2. The eggs should be poured over the squash, ricotta should be dolloped on top, and cayenne should be sprinkled on top. Bake for 20 minutes at 300 degrees Fahrenheit (149 degrees Celsius)

until the frittata is set and golden brown on top. Take the skillet out of the air fryer and slice the frittata into wedges.

Per Serving

Calories: 289 | fat: 22g | protein: 18g | carbs: 5g | fiber: 1g | sodium: 184mg

Spinach and Mushroom Mini Quiche

Prep time: 10 minutes | Cook time: 15 minutes | Serves 4
Ingredients:

- 1 tsp olive oil, plus more for spraying
- 1 cup of coarsely chopped mushrooms
- 1 cup of fresh baby spinach, shredded
- 4 eggs, beaten
- 1/2 cup of shredded Cheddar cheese
- 1/2 cup of shredded Mozzarella cheese
- 1/4 tsp salt
- 1/4 tsp black pepper

Directions:

1. Prepare 4 olive oil-sprayed silicone muffin cups of in advance.
2. One tsp of olive oil should be heated over medium heat in a medium sauté pan. Sauté the mushrooms for about three to four minutes, or until they soften.
3. Spinach should be added and cooked for 1–2 minutes, or until wilted. Don't bother with right now.
4. Mix the eggs, Cheddar cheese, mozzarella cheese, salt, and pepper in a medium Cup.
5. Blend the eggs and milk together, then stir in the mushrooms and spinach.

6. Distribute a quarter of the batter into each silicone muffin cup of.

7. Air fried the baking cups of for 5 minutes at 350 degrees Fahrenheit (177 degrees Celsius). Then, after 3–5 minutes of air frying, give the mixture in each ramekin a little stir.

Per Serving

Calories: 156 | fat: 10g | protein: 14g | carbs: 2g | fiber: 1g | sodium: 411mg

Mexican Breakfast Pepper Rings

Prep time: 5 minutes | Cook time: 10 minutes | Serves 4
Ingredients:

- Olive oil
- 1 large red, yellow, or orange bell pepper, cut into four 3/4-inch rings
- 4 eggs
- Salt and freshly ground black pepper, to taste
- 2 tbsp salsa

Directions:

1. To begin, set the temperature of the air fryer to 177 °C (350 °F). Olive oil spray should be used on a baking dish.

2. Put two pepper rings on the stovetop. The eggs should be broken into each bell pepper ring. Add salt and pepper to taste.

3. Scoop a half a spoonful of salsa and dollop it onto each egg.

4. Cookware basket goes inside air fryer. Eggs may be air-fried for 5–6 minutes for a slightly runny yolk or 8–10 minutes for a completely cooked yolk.

5. It should be done again with the other two pepper rings. Cook thoroughly and serve immediately.

Per Serving

Calories: 76 | fat: 4g | protein: 6g | carbs: 3g | fiber: 1g | sodium: 83mg

Smoky Sausage Patties

Prep time: 30 minutes | Cook time: 9 minutes | Serves 8
Ingredients:

- 1 Ib. (454 g) ground pork
- 1 tbsp coconut aminos
- 2 tbsp liquid smoke
- 1 tsp dried sage
- 1 tsp sea salt
- 1/2 tsp fennel seeds
- 1/2 tsp dried thyme
- 1/2 tsp freshly ground black pepper
- 1/4 tsp cayenne pepper

Directions:

1. Mix the pork with the liquid smoke, coconut aminos, sage, salt, fennel seeds, thyme, black pepper, and cayenne pepper in a large Cup. Mix the ingredients into the meat by working it with your hands.
2. Make 8 uniform burgers with the mixture. Put a divot in the middle of each patty with your thumb. Wrap the plastic wrap tightly around the dish containing the patties. The burgers should chill in the fridge for at least half an hour.

3. Put the patties in the air fryer in a single layer without crowding them, working in batches if required.

4. To air fry, preheat the appliance to 400 degrees Fahrenheit (204 degrees Celsius) and cook for 5 minutes. Cook the other side for another 4 minutes.

Per Serving

Calories: 70 | fat: 2g | protein: 12g | carbs: 0g | fiber: 0g | sodium: 329mg

Spinach and Feta Egg Bake

Prep time: 7 minutes | Cook time: 23 to 25 minutes | Serves 2
Ingredients:

- Avocado oil spray
- 1/3 cup of diced red onion
- 1 cup of frozen chopped spinach, thawed and drained
- 4 large eggs
- 1/4 cup of heavy cream
- Sea salt and freshly ground black pepper, to taste
- 1/4 tsp cayenne pepper
- 1/2 cup of crumbled feta cheese
- 1/4 cup of shredded Parmesan cheese

Directions:

1. Coat the bottom of a large skillet with oil spray. Place the pan with the onion in it into the air fryer's basket. Adjust the temperature of the air fryer to 350 degrees Fahrenheit (177 degrees Celsius), and bake for 7 minutes.

2. Combine the onion and spinach and sprinkle on top.

3. Whisk together the eggs, heavy cream, salt, black pepper, and cayenne in a medium Cup. Toss the veggies in this sauce.

4. Add the feta and the Parmesan on top. Put it in the oven for 16-18 minutes, or until the eggs are set and beginning to brown.

Per Serving

Calories: 366 | fat: 26g | protein: 25g | carbs: 8g | fiber: 3g | sodium: 520mg

Jalapeño Popper Egg Cups

Prep time: 10 minutes | Cook time: 10 minutes | Serves 2
Ingredients:

- 4 large eggs
- 1/4 cup of chopped pickled jalapeños
- 2 OZs (57 g) full-fat cream cheese
- 1/2 cup of shredded sharp Cheddar cheese

Directions:

1. The eggs should be beaten in a medium dish and then poured into four silicone muffin cups.

2. Combine the jalapenos, cream cheese, and Cheddar in a large microwave-safe Cup. Stir after 30 seconds in the microwave. Put about a quarter of the mixture into the middle of one of the egg cups using a spoon. Repeat with remaining mixture.

3. Fill the basket of your air fryer with egg cups. 4 Set the oven to 320 degrees Fahrenheit (160 degrees Celsius), and bake for 10 minutes. 5. Serve warm.

Per Serving

Calories: 375 | fat: 30g | protein: 23g | carbs: 3g | fiber: 0g | sodium: 445mg

Buffalo Egg Cups

Prep time: 10 minutes | Cook time: 15 minutes | Serves 2
Ingredients:

- 4 large eggs
- 2 OZs (57 g) full-fat cream cheese
- 2 tbsp buffalo sauce
- 1/2 cup of shredded sharp Cheddar cheese

Directions:

1. Separate eggs between two Cups.
2. Cream cheese, Buffalo sauce, and Cheddar should be combined in a small microwave-safe Cup. Put it in the microwave for 20 seconds and mix it up. After the eggs have been added to the ramekins, dollop some of the mixture on top.
3. The air fryer basket is where the ramekins should go. The fourth step is to bake at 320 degrees Fahrenheit (160 degrees Celsius) for 15 minutes. The fifth and final rule: serve hot.

Per Serving

Calories: 354 | fat: 29g | protein: 21g | carbs: 3g | fiber: 0g | sodium: 343mg

Portobello Eggs Benedict

Prep time: 10 minutes | Cook time: 10 to 14 minutes | Serves 2
Ingredients:

- 1 tbsp olive oil
- 2 cloves garlic, minced
- 1/4 tsp dried thyme
- 2 portobello mushrooms, stems removed and gills scraped out
- 2 Roma tomatoes, halved lengthwise
- Salt and freshly ground black pepper, to taste
- 2 large eggs
- 2 tbsp grated Pecorino Romano cheese
- 1 tbsp chopped fresh parsley, for garnish
- 1 tsp truffle oil

Directions

1. To begin, set the temperature of the air fryer to 204 degrees Fahrenheit.
2. Mix the olive oil, garlic, and thyme in a small Cup. Coat the sliced mushrooms and tomatoes with the mixture by brushing it on. Blend in some salt and freshly ground black pepper to your liking.
3. Place the veggies in the air fryer basket with the sliced sides facing up. Put an egg in the hollow of each mushroom and top with melted cheese. Prepare in an air fryer for 10–14 minutes, depending on whether you like soft or firm veggies and egg whites. Coarsely cut the tomatoes after they have cooled enough to be handled and then set them on the eggs. Prior to serving, sprinkle some chopped parsley on top and, if used, a little coating of truffle oil.

Per Serving

Calories: 189 | fat: 13g | protein: 11g | carbs: 7g | fiber: 2g | sodium: 87mg

Broccoli-Mushroom Frittata

Prep time: 10 minutes | Cook time: 20 minutes | Serves 2
Ingredients:

- 1 tbsp olive oil
- 1-1/2 cups of broccoli florets, finely chopped
- 1/2 cup of sliced brown mushrooms
- 1/4 cup of finely chopped onion
- 1/2 tsp salt
- 1/4 tsp freshly ground black pepper
- 6 eggs
- 1/4 cup of Parmesan cheese

Directions:

1. Spread the olive oil, broccoli, mushrooms, onion, salt, and pepper in a 9-by-13-inch cake pan that has a nonstick coating. Keep stirring until all of the veggies are covered with oil. Set the air fryer to 400 degrees Fahrenheit (204 degrees Celsius) with the cake pan within the basket. Cook in an air fryer for 5 minutes, or until the veggies are tender.

2. Meanwhile, mix the eggs and Parmesan in a medium Cup by whisking them together. Gently shake the pan while pouring the egg mixture in to evenly distribute the veggies. Cook for a further 15 minutes in the air fryer to set the eggs.

3. After 5 minutes in the air fryer, take the food out and let it cool down. Serve the frittata by carefully lifting it onto a platter using a silicone spatula.

Per Serving

Calories: 329 | fat: 23g | protein: 24g | carbs: 6g | fiber: 0g | sodium: 793mg

Cauliflower Avocado Toast

Prep time: 15 minutes | Cook time: 8 minutes | Serves 2
Ingredients:

- 1 (12-OZ / 340-g) steamer bag cauliflower
- 1 large egg
- 1/2 cup of shredded Mozzarella cheese
- 1 ripe medium avocado
- 1/2 tsp garlic powder
- 1/4 tsp ground black pepper

Directions:

1. Prepare cauliflower as directed on the packaging. Take out of the bag and put in a cheesecloth or dry towel to soak up the extra liquid.
2. Prepare cauliflower by placing it in a big Cup and then adding an egg and some Mozzarella cheese. Measure the inside of your air fryer basket and cut a piece of parchment paper to fit it. Make two mounds on the paper with the cauliflower mixture. Flatten the cauliflower into a 1/4-inch-thick rectangle. Put the parchment paper in the air fryer.
3. Put in an 8-minute cycle with the oven preheated to 400 degrees Fahrenheit (204 degrees Celsius). Cook the cauliflower for half the time and then flip it.
4. When the timer goes off, take the cauliflower out of the oven and let it cool for 5 minutes in the paper. Six, peel the avocado and take out the seed. Remove the pulp, set it in a medium Cup,

and mash it with the aforementioned seasonings. Apply the spread on the cauliflower. Quickly dish it up.

Per Serving

Calories: 321 | fat: 22g | protein: 16g | carbs: 19g | fiber: 10g | sodium: 99mg

Morning Buzz Iced Coffee

Prep time: 10 minutes | Cook time: 0 minutes | Serves 1
Ingredients:

- 1 cup of freshly brewed strong black coffee, cooled slightly
- 1 tbsp extra-virgin olive oil
- 1 tbsp half-and-half or heavy cream
- 1 tsp MCT oil
- 1/8 tsp almond extract
- 1/8 tsp ground cinnamon

Directions:

1. Place the coffee in a blender or a large glass and let it cool slightly.
2. Add the almond extract, cinnamon, MCT oil, half-and-half, if using, and olive oil. 3. Combine thoroughly so that there is no trace of lumps left. Relax with a hot beverage.

Per Serving

Calories: 124 | fat: 14g | protein: 0g | carbs: 0g | fiber: 0g | sodium: 5mg

Lemon–Olive Oil Breakfast Cakes with Berry Syrup

Prep time: 5 minutes | Cook time: 10 minutes | Serves 4
Ingredients:

For the Pancakes:
- 1 cup of almond flour
- 1 tsp baking powder
- 1/4 tsp salt
- 6 tbsp extra-virgin olive oil, divided
- 2 large eggs
- Zest and juice of 1 lemon
- 1/2 tsp almond or vanilla extract

For the Berry Sauce:
- 1 cup of frozen mixed berries
- 1 tbsp water or lemon juice, plus more if needed
- 1/2 tsp vanilla extract

Directions:

Make the Pancakes:

1. Mix the almond flour, baking powder, and salt in a large Cup and whisk to combine and remove any lumps.
2. Whisk in the eggs, almond essence, lemon zest, lemon juice, and the remaining 4 tbsp of olive oil.
3. Cook 4 pancakes at a time using 2 tbsp of batter each pancake in a big skillet coated with 1 tbsp of olive oil heated over medium. After 4–5 minutes, when bubbles start to develop, turn the pancake. Return to the stove for another three minutes of cooking time. Use the remaining 1 tbsp olive oil and batter for another round.

Make the Berry Sauce:

1. Warm the frozen berries, water, and vanilla essence in a small saucepan over medium heat for 3 to 4 minutes, until bubbling; if necessary, thin with more water. Mash the berries with a spoon or fork and whisk them till smooth.

Per Serving

Calories: 381 | fat: 35g | protein: 8g | carbs: 12g | fiber: 4g | sodium: 183mg

Greek Egg and Tomato Scramble

Prep time: 10 minutes | Cook time: 25 minutes | Serves 4
Ingredients:

- 1/4 cup of extra-virgin olive oil, divided
- 1-1/2 cups of chopped fresh tomatoes
- 1/4 cup of finely minced red onion
- 2 garlic cloves, minced
- 1/2 tsp dried oregano or 1 to 2 tbsp chopped fresh oregano
- 1/2 tsp dried thyme or 1 to 2 tbsp chopped fresh thyme
- 8 large eggs
- 1/2 tsp salt
- 1/4 tsp freshly ground black pepper
- 3/4 cup of crumbled feta cheese
- 1/4 cup of chopped fresh mint leaves

Directions:

2. Olive oil should be heated over medium heat in a big skillet. Ten to twelve minutes after adding the tomatoes and red onion, the tomatoes should be cooked through and tender.

3. For another 2–4 minutes of cooking, when the liquid has decreased and the flavors have melded, add the garlic, oregano, and thyme.
4. Stir the eggs, salt, and pepper together in a medium Cup.
5. Throw the eggs into the pan, turn the heat down to low, and scramble them for about four minutes, while continually stirring with a spatula, until they are firm and creamy. Take the pan off the burner and toss in the mint and feta cheese; serve hot.

Per Serving

Calories: 355 | fat: 29g | protein: 17g | carbs: 6g | fiber: 1g | sodium: 695mg

Mashed Chickpea, Feta, and Avocado Toast

Prep time: 10 minutes |Cook time: 0 minutes| Serves: 4
Ingredients:

- 1 (15-OZ / 425-g) can chickpeas, drained and rinsed
- 1 avocado, pitted
- 1/2 cup of diced feta cheese (about 2 OZs / 57 g)
- 2 tbsp freshly squeezed lemon juice or 1 tbsp orange juice
- 1/2 tsp freshly ground black pepper
- 4 pieces multigrain toast
- 2 tbsp honey

Directions:

1. Prepare a sizable basin for the chickpeas. Put the flesh of the avocados in the basin.
2. To make a spreadable mixture, mash all the ingredients together with a potato masher or a big fork. It need not be flawless.

3. Mix in the lemon juice, feta, and pepper.

4. Slice the bread in half and spoon the mash evenly over all four slices. Serve with a honey drizzle.

Per Serving

Calories: 301 | fat: 14g | protein: 12g | carbs: 35g | fiber: 11g | sodium: 450mg

Quickie Honey Nut Granola

Prep time: 10 minutes |Cook time: 20 minutes| Serves: 6
Ingredients:

- 2-1/2 cups of regular rolled oats
- 1/3 cup of coarsely chopped almonds
- 1/8 tsp kosher or sea salt
- 1/2 tsp ground cinnamon
- 1/2 cup of chopped dried apricots
- 2 tbsp ground flaxseed
- 1/4 cup of honey
- 1/4 cup of extra-virgin olive oil
- 2 tbsp vanilla extract

Directions:

1. Set oven temperature to 325 degrees F (165 degrees C). Use parchment paper to line a large, rimmed baking sheet.

2. Mix the oats, almonds, salt, and cinnamon in a big pan. Toast the nuts in 6 minutes over medium heat, stirring often.

3. While the oat mixture toasts, prepare the apricots by combining them with flaxseed, honey, and oil in a microwave-safe dish. Warm it in the microwave for approximately a minute on high, or until it is extremely hot and starts to boil. (Alternatively,

bring these ingredients to a simmer in a small saucepan over medium heat for approximately 3 minutes.)

4. Blend in the vanilla to the honey and drizzle it over the oats in the pan. Incorporate well by stirring.

5. The granola should be evenly distributed on the baking sheet. Put it in the oven and brown it a little bit, maybe 15 minutes. Take it out of the oven and let it cool down.

6. The granola may be kept in an airtight jar for up to two weeks in the fridge (if it lasts that long!).

Per Serving

Calories: 449 | fat: 17g | protein: 13g | carbs: 64g | fiber: 9g | sodium: 56mg

Mediterranean Fruit Bulgur Breakfast Cup

Prep time: 5 minutes |Cook time: 15 minutes| Serves: 6
Ingredients:

- 1-1/2 cups of uncooked bulgur
- 2 cups of 2% milk
- 1 cup of water
- 1/2 tsp ground cinnamon
- 2 cups of frozen (or fresh, pitted) dark sweet cherries
- 8 dried (or fresh) figs, chopped
- 1/2 cup of chopped almonds
- 1/4 cup of loosely packed fresh mint, chopped
- Warm 2% milk, for serving

Directions:

1. Stir the bulgur, milk, water, and cinnamon together in a medium pot. Give it a quick stir, and then bring it to a boil. Cover and

simmer over low heat, stirring occasionally, for 10 minutes, or until the liquid is absorbed.

2. Do not defrost the frozen cherries before adding them to the pan along with the figs and almonds. The frozen cherries and figs may be thawed in the hot bulgur by stirring thoroughly, covering the pot for a minute, and then removing the lid. Blend with some fresh mint.

3. Divide among Cups for serving. If you like, accompany with warm milk. It's also delicious when served cold.

Per Serving

Calories: 273 | fat: 7g | protein: 10g | carbs: 48g | fiber: 8g | sodium: 46mg

Marinara Eggs with Parsley

Prep time: 5 minutes |Cook time: 15 minutes| Serves: 6
Ingredients:

- 1 tbsp extra-virgin olive oil
- 1 cup of chopped onion (about 1/2 medium onion) sp
- 2 garlic cloves, minced (about 1 tsp)
- 2 (141/2-OZ / 411-g) cans Italian diced tomatoes, undrained, no salt added
- 6 large eggs
- 1/2 cup of chopped fresh flat-leaf (Italian) parsley
- Crusty Italian bread and grated Parmesan or Romano cheese, for serving
  Directions:

1. Oil should be heated in a big pan over moderate heat. Stirring periodically, sauté the onion for 5 minutes. Put in the garlic and let it sizzle for a minute.

2. Add the tomatoes and their juice to the onion mixture and let it simmer for about 3 minutes, or until it begins to bubble. Crack an egg into a small custard cup of coffee mug as you wait for the tomato mixture to boil.

3. Turn the heat down to medium when the tomato mixture begins to boil. Then, form six wells in the tomato mixture using a big spoon. Carefully pour the first cracked egg into one indentation, then continue with the other eggs, breaking them one at a time into the custard cup and pouring them one at a time into each indentation. Cover the pan and cook the eggs for 6 to 7 minutes, or until they reach the desired doneness (about 6 minutes for soft-cooked, 7 minutes for harder cooked).

4. Serve with bread and grated cheese on the side, and sprinkle with parsley before serving.

Per Serving

Calories: 127 | fat: 7g | protein: 8g | carbs: 8g | fiber: 2g | sodium: 82mg

Homemade Pumpkin Parfait

Prep time: 5 minutes | Cook time: 0 minutes | Serves 4
Ingredients:

- 1 (15-OZ / 425-g) can pure pumpkin purée
- 4 tbsp honey, additional to taste
- 1 tsp pumpkin pie spice
- 1/4 tsp ground cinnamon

- 2 cups of plain, unsweetened, full-fat Greek yogurt
- 1 cup of honey granola

Directions:

1. Combine the pumpkin puree, honey, pumpkin pie spice, and cinnamon in a large Cup and stir to combine. Chill for at least two hours after covering and refrigerating.
2. Make the parfaits by layering a quarter cup of pumpkin mix, a quarter cup of yogurt, and a quarter cup of granola into each cup. Layers of pumpkin and Greek yogurt are repeated, and then honey granola is sprinkled on top.

Per Serving

Calories: 264 | fat: 9g | protein: 15g | carbs: 35g | fiber: 6g | sodium: 90mg

South of the Coast Sweet Potato Toast

Prep time: 5 minutes | Cook time: 15 minutes | Serves 4
Ingredients:

- 2 plum tomatoes, halved
- 6 tbsp extra-virgin olive oil, divided
- Salt
- Freshly ground black pepper
- 2 large sweet potatoes, sliced lengthwise
- 1 cup of fresh spinach
- 8 medium asparagus, trimmed
- 4 large cooked eggs or egg substitute
- 1 cup of arugula
- 4 tbsp pesto

- 4 tbsp shredded Asiago cheese

Directions:

1. Turn the oven temperature up to 450F (235C).
2. Spread the plum tomato halves on a baking sheet and drizzle with 2 tsp.. of olive oil; sprinkle with salt and pepper. After about 15 minutes in the oven, take the tomatoes and set them aside to cool.
3. Spread the sweet potato slices in a single layer on a baking sheet, coat each side with approximately 2 tsp.. of oil, and season with salt and pepper. In a preheated oven, bake the sweet potato slices for 15 minutes, turning once after 7 minutes. Take out of the oven.
4. The fresh spinach may be sautéed in a skillet or sauté pan with the remaining 2 tsp.. of olive oil over medium heat until it is barely wilted. Take out of the pan and place on a paper towel-lined plate to cool. Sauté the asparagus in the same pan, stirring occasionally. Place on a plate lined with paper towels.
5. Arrange the spinach and asparagus among the grilled sweet potato pieces on individual plates. On top of the cooked spinach and asparagus, place one egg. Top with arugula, about a quarter cup's worth. To finish, add 1 tsp. of pesto and 1 tsp. of cheese. Pair with a roasted plum tomato for each serving.

Per Serving

Calories: 441 | fat: 35g | protein: 13g | carbs: 23g | fiber: 4g | sodium: 481mg

Honey-Balsamic Salmon

Prep time: 5 minutes | Cook time: 8 minutes | Serves 2
Ingredients:

- Oil, for spraying
- 2 (6-OZ / 170-g) salmon fillets
- 1/4 cup of balsamic vinegar
- 2 tbsp honey
- 2 tbsp red pepper flakes
- 2 tbsp olive oil
- 1/2 tsp salt
- 1/4 tsp freshly ground black pepper

Directions:

1. Spray oil sparingly into the air fryer basket and line it with parchment paper.
2. Prepare a basket for the salmon.
3. To make the dressing, combine the balsamic vinegar, honey, red pepper flakes, olive oil, salt, and black pepper in a small Cup and whisk until smooth. Salmon should be coated with the mixture.
4. Roast at 390 degrees Fahrenheit (199 degrees Celsius) for 7 to 8 minutes, or until the interior temperature reaches 145 degrees Fahrenheit (63 degrees Celsius). Start serving right now.

Per Serving
Calories: 353 | fat: 12g | protein: 35g | carbs: 24g | fiber: 1g | sodium: 590mg

Blackened Red Snapper

Prep time: 13 minutes | Cook time: 8 to 10 minutes | Serves 4
Ingredients:

- 1-1/2 tbsp black pepper
- 1/4 tsp thyme
- 1/4 tsp garlic powder
- 1/8 tsp cayenne pepper
- 1 tsp olive oil
- 4 (4-OZ / 113-g) red snapper fillet portions, skin on
- 4 thin slices lemon
- Cooking spray

Directions:

1. Create a paste by combining the oil and spices. Coat both sides of the fish with the rub.
2. Before placing the snapper steaks skin-side down in the air fryer basket, spray the basket with nonstick cooking spray.
3. Put a slice of lemon on top of each fish fillet.
4. Roast for 8-10 minutes at 390F (199C). When done, the fish will not flake, but the middle should be a solid white.

Per Serving
Calories: 128 | fat: 3g | protein: 23g | carbs: 1g | fiber: 1g | sodium: 73mg

Chilean Sea Bass with Olive Relish

Prep time: 10 minutes | Cook time: 10 minutes | Serves 2
Ingredients:

- Olive oil spray
- 2 (6-OZ / 170-g) Chilean sea bass fillets or other firm-fleshed white fish
- 3 tbsp extra-virgin olive oil
- 1/2 tsp ground cumin
- 1/2 tsp kosher salt
- 1/2 tsp black pepper
- 1/3 cup of pitted green olives, diced
- 1/4 cup of finely diced onion
- 1 tsp chopped capers

Directions:

1. Apply olive oil spray to the basket of the air fryer. Drizzle the fillets with the olive oil and sprinkle with the cumin, salt, and pepper. Place the fish in the air fryer basket. Set the air fryer to 325°F (163°C) for 10 minutes, or until the fish flakes easily with a fork.
2. At the same time, combine the olives, onion, and capers in a separate small Cup and mix to combine.
3. Arrange the relish on top of the fish before serving.

Per Serving
Calories: 379 | fat: 26g | protein: 32g | carbs: 3g | fiber: 1g | sodium: 581mg

Black Cod with Grapes and Kale

Prep time: 10 minutes | Cook time: 15 minutes | Serves 2
Ingredients:

- 2 (6- to 8-OZ / 170- to 227-g) fillets of black cod
- Salt and freshly ground black pepper, to taste
- Olive oil
- 1 cup of grapes, halved
- 1 small bulb fennel, sliced 1/4-inch thick
- 1/2 cup of pecans
- 3 cups of shredded kale
- 2 tbsp white balsamic vinegar or white wine vinegar
- 2 tbsp extra-virgin olive oil

Directions:

1. Air fryer temperature should be set at 400 degrees Fahrenheit (204 degrees Celsius).
2. Salt and pepper the cod fillets, and then apply a light coating of olive oil by drizzling, brushing, or spraying. Flip the fish over so that the skin is facing up in the air fryer basket. Take 10 minutes to air fry.
3. Fish fillets may be rested after cooking by moving them to a platter and tenting them lightly with foil.
4. Sprinkle some salt and pepper on the grapes, fennel, and pecans before tossing them in a dish with some olive oil. Put the grapes, fennel, and pecans in the air fryer's basket and cook them at 400 degrees Fahrenheit (204 degrees Celsius) for 5 minutes, while shaking the basket once.
5. Mix the kale with the grapes, fennel, and pecans in a Cup. Season the kale with salt and pepper, then dress it with balsamic vinegar and olive oil. Serve it with the salmon.

Per Serving
Calories: 509 | fat: 33g | protein: 31g | carbs: 28g | fiber: 8g | sodium: 587mg

Maple Balsamic Glazed Salmon

Prep time: 5 minutes | Cook time: 10 minutes | Serves 4
Ingredients:

- 4 (6-OZ / 170-g) fillets of salmon
- Salt and freshly ground black pepper, to taste
- Vegetable oil
- 1/4 cup of pure maple syrup
- 3 tbsp balsamic vinegar
- 1 tsp Dijon mustard

Directions:

1. Air fryer temperature should be set at 400 degrees Fahrenheit (204 degrees Celsius).
2. Use plenty of salt and freshly ground black pepper when seasoning the fish. Prepare the air fryer by spraying or brushing the bottom of the basket with vegetable oil, and then adding the salmon fillets. Set the air fryer to 375 degrees and cook the fish for 5 minutes.
3. While the salmon is air-frying, make the sauce by heating the maple syrup, balsamic vinegar, and Dijon mustard together in a small pot. While the fish is in the oven, simmer the mixture. Keep an eye on it as it thickens to prevent it from burning.
4. The salmon fillets will need an extra 5 minutes in the air fryer after being glazed. When the salmon is done, it should feel firm to the touch and the glaze should have browned attractively on

top. Brush some more glaze on top, then remove and serve with rice and vegetables or a fresh green salad.

Per Serving
Calories: 279 | fat: 8g | protein: 35g | carbs: 15g | fiber: 0g | sodium: 146mg

Sesame-Crusted Tuna Steak

Prep time: 5 minutes | Cook time: 8 minutes | Serves 2
Ingredients:

- 2 (6-OZ / 170-g) tuna steaks
- 1 tbsp coconut oil, melted
- 1/2 tsp garlic powder
- 2 tbsp white sesame seeds
- 2 tbsp black sesame seeds

Directions

1. Coconut oil and garlic powder should be used to coat each tuna steak.
2. The tuna steaks are coated in sesame seeds by pressing them into the seeds in a big basin. Toss some tuna steaks into the basket of your air fryer.
3. Air fried at 400 degrees Fahrenheit (204 degrees Celsius) for 8 minutes.
4. Approximately halfway through cooking, turn the steaks over. 145 degrees Fahrenheit (63 degrees Celsius) is the magic number for well-done steaks. Hold back the heat.

Per Serving
Calories: 281 | fat: 11g | protein: 43g | carbs: 1g | fiber: 1g | sodium: 80mg

Mediterranean-Style Cod

Prep time: 5 minutes | Cook time: 12 minutes | Serves 4
Ingredients:

- 4 (6-OZ / 170-g) cod fillets
- 3 tbsp fresh lemon juice
- 1 tbsp olive oil
- 1/4 tsp salt
- 6 cherry tomatoes, halved
- 1/4 cup of pitted and sliced kalamata olives

Directions:

1. Do not butter a 9-inch round baking dish; add the fish to the dish. Cod with olive oil and fresh lemon juice. Toss some salt on it. Fill the empty spaces between the fillets with tomato slices and olives.
2. Put the dish in the basket of the air fryer. Bake the fish for 12 minutes at 350 degrees Fahrenheit (177 degrees Celsius), rotating once halfway through. When done, fillets will have an internal temperature of at least 145 degrees Fahrenheit (63 degrees Celsius), be lightly browned, and flake readily. Hold back the heat.

Per Serving
Calories: 186 | fat: 5g | protein: 31g | carbs: 2g | fiber: 1g | sodium: 300mg

Cucumber and Salmon Salad

Prep time: 10 minutes | Cook time: 8 to 10 minutes | Serves 2
Ingredients:

- 1 Ib. (454 g) salmon fillet
- 1-1/2 tbsp olive oil, divided
- 1 tbsp sherry vinegar
- 1 tbsp capers, rinsed and drained
- 1 seedless cucumber, thinly sliced
- 1/4 Vidalia onion, thinly sliced
- 2 tbsp chopped fresh parsley
- Salt and freshly ground black pepper, to taste
  Directions:

1. Air fryer temperature should be set at 400 degrees Fahrenheit (204 degrees Celsius).
2. Rub half of the tbsp of olive oil all over the fish. Air fried the salmon skin-side down for 8-10 minutes, or until it is opaque and flakes readily when tested with a fork. Place the salmon on a platter and refrigerate until cold. Carefully peel off the skin and flake the fish into little pieces.
3. Combine the remaining 1 tbsp olive oil with the vinegar in a small Cup and whisk until smooth. Mix in the capers, diced cucumber, diced onion, and chopped parsley. Add salt and freshly ground black pepper to taste. Softly toss to evenly distribute the coating. In any case, serve right away or store in the fridge for up to 4 hours covered.

Per Serving
Calories: 399 | fat: 20g | protein: 47g | carbs: 4g | fiber: 1g | sodium: 276mg

Tuna Steaks with Olive Tapenade

Prep time: 10 minutes | Cook time: 10 minutes | Serves 4
Ingredients:

- 4 (6-OZ / 170-g) ahi tuna steaks
- 1 tbsp olive oil
- Salt and freshly ground black pepper, to taste
- 1/2 lemon, sliced into 4 wedges
- Olive Tapenade:
- 1/2 cup of pitted kalamata olives
- 1 tbsp olive oil
- 1 tbsp chopped fresh parsley
- 1 clove garlic
- 2 tbsp red wine vinegar
- 1 tsp capers, drained

Directions:

1. Make sure your air fryer is at 400 degrees Fahrenheit.
2. Apply half the tsp. of olive oil to the fish and rub it all over. Cooked the salmon in an air fryer, skin side down, for 8-10 minutes, or until it was opaque throughout and flaked easily with a fork. Make the salmon into a cold appetizer by placing it on a platter and chilling it in the fridge. It's best to remove the skin slowly and carefully before flaking the fish.
3. Whisk together the remaining 1 tbsp of olive oil and the vinegar in a small Cup. Combine the chopped parsley, onion, cucumber, and capers. To taste, season with salt and freshly ground black pepper. Using a gentle tossing motion, evenly distribute the coating. If not serving right away, cover and place in the refrigerator for up to 4 hours.

Per Serving

Calories: 269 | fat: 9g | protein: 42g | carbs: 2g | fiber: 1g | sodium: 252mg

Marinated Swordfish Skewers

Prep time: 30 minutes | Cook time: 6 to 8 minutes | Serves 4
Ingredients:

- 1 Ib. (454 g) filleted swordfish
- 1/4 cup of avocado oil
- 2 tbsp freshly squeezed lemon juice
- 1 tbsp minced fresh parsley
- 2 tbsp Dijon mustard
- Sea salt and freshly ground black pepper, to taste
- 3 OZs (85 g) cherry tomatoes

Directions:

1. Separate any residual bones from the fish before cutting it into 11/2-inch cubes.
2. Oil, lemon juice, chopped parsley, and Dijon mustard are combined in a large basin and whisked together. Sprinkle with salt and pepper to taste. Toss the fish in the sauce to coat it. Marinating the fish for 30 minutes in the fridge is a great idea.
3. Toss the marinade and fish. Skewer the fish and cherry tomatoes in alternating fashion on four skewers.
4. Temperature of 400 degrees Fahrenheit (204 degrees C) in the air fryer is recommended. Just throw the skewers into the air fryer and cook them for three minutes. To ensure the fish is cooked all the way through, use an instant-read thermometer to check its temperature after 3 to 5 minutes of cooking.

Per Serving
Calories: 291 | fat: 21g | protein: 23g | carbs: 2g | fiber: 0g | sodium: 121mg

Salmon with Provolone Cheese

Prep time: 5 minutes | Cook time: 15 minutes | Serves 4
Ingredients:

- 1 Ib. (454 g) salmon fillet, chopped
- 2 OZs (57 g) Provolone, grated
- 1 tsp avocado oil
- 1/4 tsp ground paprika

Directions

1. Salmon fillets coated with avocado oil and cooked in an air fryer.
2. Then, after baking, sprinkle the Provolone cheese and crushed paprika over the fish.
3. Prepare the fish for 15 minutes at 360 degrees Fahrenheit (182 degrees Celsius).

Per Serving
Calories: 204 | fat: 10g | protein: 27g | carbs: 0g | fiber: 0g | sodium: 209mg

Parmesan Mackerel with Coriander

Prep time: 10 minutes | Cook time: 7 minutes | Serves 2
Ingredients:

- 12 OZs (340 g) mackerel fillet
- 2 OZs (57 g) Parmesan, grated
- 1 tsp ground coriander
- 1 tbsp olive oil

Direction:

1. Add the mackerel fillets to the air fryer basket and drizzle with olive oil.

2. Sprinkle some ground coriander and grated Parmesan cheese over the fish.
3. Prepare the fish for 7 minutes at 390 degrees Fahrenheit (199 degrees Celsius).

Per Serving
Calories: 522 | fat: 39g | protein: 42g | carbs: 1g | fiber: 0g | sodium: 544mg

Rosemary-Lemon Snapper Baked in Parchment

Prep time: 15 minutes | Cook time: 15 minutes | Serves 4
Ingredients:

- 1-1/4 Ib.s (567 g) fresh red snapper fillet, cut into two equal pieces
- 2 lemons, thinly sliced
- 6 to 8 sprigs fresh rosemary, stems removed or 1 to 2 tbsp dried rosemary
- 1/2 cup of extra-virgin olive oil
- 6 garlic cloves, thinly sliced
- 1 tsp salt
- 1/2 tsp freshly ground black pepper

Direction:

1. Prepare a 425F (220C) oven.
2. Spread out on the kitchen counter two big pieces of parchment paper (each one should be nearly twice the size of the fish). Put a single piece of fish in the middle of each page.
3. Prepare the fish and then garnish with lemon slices and fresh rosemary.
4. Mix the garlic, olive oil, salt, and pepper in a small Cup. Spread the oil all over the fish.

5. Place a second big sheet of parchment on top of the fish and, beginning with a long side, fold it up to within about an inch of the fish. The same procedure should be followed, clockwise, on the other sides. For extra safety, double-fold each corner inward.
6. After 10 to 12 minutes in the oven, remove the paper pouches to check the fish.

Per Serving
Calories: 399 | fat: 29g | protein: 30g | carbs: 5g | fiber: 1g | sodium: 584mg

Shrimp in Creamy Pesto over Zoodles

Prep time: 10 minutes | Cook time: 10 minutes | Serves 4
Ingredients:

- 1 Ib. (454 g) peeled and deveined fresh shrimp
- Salt
- Freshly ground black pepper
- 2 tbsp extra-virgin olive oil
- 1/2 small onion, slivered
- 8 OZs (227 g) store-bought jarred pesto
- 3/4 cup of crumbled goat or feta cheese, plus more for serving
- 6 cups of zucchini noodles (from about 2 large zucchini), for serving
- 1/4 cup of chopped flat-leaf Italian parsley, for garnish

Direction:

1. Put the shrimp in a Cup and season with salt and pepper.
2. Olive oil should be heated over medium-high heat in a large pan. The onion should take around 5–6 minutes to get yellow when sautéed.
3. Turn the heat down to low, then stir in the pesto and cheese until the cheese melts and the two ingredients are well combined.

Shrimp should be added at the very end and the sauce should be simmering. Cover the pot and turn the heat back down to low. And for another 3–4 minutes, until the shrimp are pink and fully cooked.

4. Garnish with chopped parsley and more crumbled cheese, then serve warm over zucchini noodles.

Per Serving

Calories: 608 | fat: 49g | protein: 37g | carbs: 9g | fiber: 3g | sodium: 564mg

Salmon with Tarragon-Dijon Sauce

Prep time: 5 minutes | Cook time: 15 minutes | Serves 4
Ingredients:

- 1-1/4 Ib. (567 g) salmon fillet, cut into 4 equal pieces
- 1/4 cup of avocado oil mayonnaise
- 1/4 cup of Dijon or stone-ground mustard
- Zest and juice of 1/2 lemon
- 2 tbsp chopped fresh tarragon or 1 to 2 tbsp dried tarragon
- 1/2 tsp salt
- 1/4 tsp freshly ground black pepper
- 4 tbsp extra-virgin olive oil, for serving

  Direction:

1. Prepare a 425F (220C) oven. Get some parchment paper and line a baking pan.
2. Cook the salmon in the oven with the skin side down.
3. Mix the mayonnaise, mustard, lemon rind and juice, tarragon, salt, and pepper in a small Cup. Evenly spread the sauce mixture on top of the salmon.
4. Bake for 10–12 minutes, depending on the thickness of the salmon, until the top is browned and the center is just beginning

to turn translucent. Take out of the oven and cool on the baking sheet for 10 minutes. When ready to serve, add 1 tsp. of olive oil to each fillet.

Per Serving
Calories: 343 | fat: 23g | protein: 30g | carbs: 4g | fiber: 1g | sodium: 585mg

Salmon with Lemon-Garlic Mashed Cauliflower

Prep time: 15 minutes | Cook time: 10 minutes | Serves 4
Ingredients:

- 2 tbsp extra-virgin olive oil
- 4 garlic cloves, peeled and smashed
- 1/2 cup of chicken or vegetable broth
- 3/4 tsp table salt, divided
- 1 large head cauliflower (3 Ib. / 1.4 kg), cored and cut into 2-inch florets
- 4 (6-OZ / 170-g) skinless salmon fillets, 1 1/2 inches thick
- 1/2 tsp Ras El hangout
- 1/2 tsp grated lemon zest
- 3 scallions, sliced thin
- 1 tbsp sesame seeds, toasted

Direction

1. Instant Pot's highest sauté setting should be used to prepare the oil and garlic until the garlic is aromatic and light golden brown, which should take around 3 minutes. After the pressure cooker has been turned off, add the broth and a pinch of salt and mix well. Layer cauliflower evenly in the pot.
2. Make a sling from a 16-by-6-inch piece of aluminum foil. Skin side down in the middle of the sling, sprinkle the flesh side with the Ras El hangout and the remaining 1/2 tsp of salt. Place the

sling's thin edges along the insert's sides, then drop the salmon into the Instant Pot on top of the cauliflower. Seal the container and turn off the pressure release valve. To cook in two minutes using high pressure, choose that option.

3. Quickly release pressure by switching off the Instant Pot. Remove the lid slowly and carefully so that the steam may escape in a safe direction. Bring the fish to the big platter using the sling. Wrap in foil and rest while you finish cooking the cauliflower.

4. Reduce the size of any big pieces of cauliflower by mashing the mixture with a potato masher. When cooking cauliflower, use the highest sauté setting and cook it for 3 minutes, turning often, or until it has thickened significantly. Salt and pepper to taste, then stir in lemon zest. Serve the salmon and cauliflower with scallions and sesame seeds on the side.

Per Serving
Calories: 480 | fat: 31g | protein: 38g | carbs: 9g | fiber: 3g | sodium: 650mg

Salmon with Garlicky Broccoli Rabe and White Beans

Prep time: 20 minutes | Cook time: 10 minutes | Serves 4
Ingredients:

- 2 tbsp extra-virgin olive oil, plus extra for drizzling
- 4 garlic cloves, sliced thin
- 1/2 cup of chicken or vegetable broth
- 1/4 tsp red pepper flakes
- 1 lemon, sliced 1/4 inch thick, plus lemon wedges for serving

- 4 (6-OZ / 170-g) skinless salmon fillets, 1 1/2 inches thick
- 1/2 tsp table salt
- 1/4 tsp pepper
- 1 Ib. (454 g) broccoli rabe, trimmed and cut into 1-inch pieces
- 1 (15-OZ / 425-g) can cannellini beans, rinsed

Direction:

1. Instant Pot's highest sauté setting should be used to prepare the oil and garlic until the garlic is aromatic and light golden brown, which should take around 3 minutes. Put the garlic on a platter lined with paper towels, season with salt, and leave aside. Stop the Instant Pot cooking process and add the broth and pepper flakes.

2. Make a sling from a 16-by-6-inch piece of aluminum foil. Place lemon slices in the middle of the sling in two rows, across the width. Fish should be salted and peppered on the flesh side before being placed skin-side down on top of lemon slices. Salmon should be lowered into the Instant Pot using the sling, with the thin edges of the sling resting on the insert's sides. Seal the container and turn off the pressure release valve. Choose the pressure-cooking mode and set the timer for 3 minutes.

3. Quickly release pressure by switching off the Instant Pot. Remove the lid slowly and carefully so that the steam may escape in a safe direction. Bring the fish to the big platter using the sling. To rest while you make the broccoli rabe combination, tent with foil.

4. Mix in the beans and broccoli rabe to the cooking liquid, cover, and simmer for 5 minutes on high sauté until the broccoli rabe is cooked. Put in as much salt and pepper as you want. Salmon fillets should be lifted and tipped gently with a spatula to allow lemon slices to fall off. Garnish individual servings of the fish

with garlic chips and a drizzle of additional oil before serving with the broccoli rabe combination and lemon wedges.

Per Serving

Calories: 510 | fat: 30g | protein: 43g | carbs: 15g | fiber: 6g | sodium: 650mg

Salmon with Wild Rice and Orange Salad

Prep time: 20 minutes | Cook time: 18 minutes | Serves 4
Ingredients:

- 1 cup of wild rice, picked over and rinsed
- 3 tbsp extra-virgin olive oil, divided
- 11/2 tsp table salt, for cooking rice
- 2 oranges, plus 1/8 tsp grated orange zest
- 4 (6-OZ / 170-g) skinless salmon fillets, 11/2 inches thick
- 1 tsp ground dried Aleppo pepper
- 1/2 tsp table salt
- 1 small shallot, minced
- 1 tbsp red wine vinegar
- 2 tbsp Dijon mustard
- 1 tsp honey
- 2 carrots, peeled and shredded
- 1/4 cup of chopped fresh mint

Direction:

1. The Instant Pot may be used to cook the rice by adding 6 cups of water, 1 tsp. of oil, and 1 1/2 tsp.. of salt. Seal the container and turn off the pressure release valve. Click the pressure cooker's high setting and set the timer for 15 minutes. After 15 minutes, turn Instant Pot off and let pressure to release on its own. Carefully remove the lid and let the steam flow away from you

after a quick pressure release. Remove the rice from the heat and put it aside to cool. Use paper towels to scrub the stovetop.

2. The Instant Pot should be filled with half a cup of water. Make a sling from a 16-by-6-inch piece of aluminum foil. Orange shingles sliced 1/4 inch thick, laid down in three rows across the sling's middle. After seasoning the flesh side of the salmon with Aleppo pepper and 1/2 tsp salt, place the fillets skin-side down on a bed of orange segments. Salmon should be lowered into the Instant Pot using the sling, with the thin edges of the sling resting on the insert's sides. Seal the container and turn off the pressure release valve. Choose the pressure-cooking mode and set the timer for 3 minutes.

3. While doing so, remove the peel and pith from the remaining orange. Cut orange in half lengthwise, then crosswise into thin slices. In a large Cup, combine the remaining 2 tsp.. of oil with the shallot, vinegar, mustard, honey, and orange zest. Stir in orange pieces, carrots, mint, and rice. Put in as much salt and pepper as you want.

4. Quickly release pressure by switching off the Instant Pot. Remove the lid slowly and carefully so that the steam may escape in a safe direction. Bring the fish to the big platter using the sling. With a spatula, carefully raise and turn the fillets to dislodge the orange slices. Toss some salmon with some salad.

Per Serving

Calories: 690 | fat: 34g | protein: 43g | carbs: 51g | fiber: 5g | sodium: 770mg

Cod with Warm Beet and Arugula Salad

Prep time: 15 minutes | Cook time: 8 minutes | Serves 4
Ingredients:

- 1/4 cup of extra-virgin olive oil, divided, plus extra for drizzling
- 1 shallot, sliced thin
- 2 garlic cloves, minced
- 1-1/2 Ib. (680 g) small beets, scrubbed, trimmed, and cut into 1/2-inch wedges
- 1/2 cup of chicken or vegetable broth
- 1 tbsp dukkah, plus extra for sprinkling
- 1/4 tsp table salt
- 4 (6-OZ / 170-g) skinless cod fillets, 11/2 inches thick
- 1 tbsp lemon juice
- 2 OZs (57 g) baby arugula

Direction:

1. One tbsp of oil should be heated in the Instant Pot until it shimmers using the highest sauté setting. Stir in the shallot and simmer for 2 minutes, or until it has softened. Add the garlic and stir for approximately 30 seconds, or until the aroma is released. Combine beets and stock and mix well. Seal the container and turn off the pressure release valve. Choose the pressure-cooking mode and set the timer for 3 minutes. Quickly release pressure by switching off the Instant Pot. Remove the lid slowly and carefully so that the steam may escape in a safe direction.

2. Make a sling from a 16-by-6-inch piece of aluminum foil. Brush the fish with the oil mixture that was made by combining 2 tbsp of olive oil with dukkah and salt in a basin. Lay the fish fillets skin side down in the middle of the sling. Put the cod into the Instant Pot using the sling, with the thin edges of the sling

resting on the insert's sides. Seal the container and turn off the pressure release valve. To cook in two minutes using high pressure, choose that option.

3. Quickly release pressure by switching off the Instant Pot. Remove the lid slowly and carefully so that the steam may escape in a safe direction. Move the fish to the big platter using the sling. Rest while you finish making the beet salad by tenting it with foil.

4. In a large dish, mix the remaining 1 tsp. of oil with the lemon juice. Place beets in the basin containing the oil and vinegar mixture using a slotted spoon. Incorporate the arugula and mix everything together gently. Put in as much salt and pepper as you want. Sprinkle more dukkah and oil over individual servings of fish and salad before serving.

per Serving
Calories: 340 | fat: 16g | protein: 33g | carbs: 14g | fiber: 4g | sodium: 460mg

Braised Striped Bass with Zucchini and Tomatoes

Prep time: 20 minutes | Cook time: 16 minutes | Serves 4
Ingredients:

- 2 tbsp extra-virgin olive oil, divided, plus extra for drizzling
- 3 zucchini (8 OZs / 227 g each), halved lengthwise and sliced 1/4 inch thick
- 1 onion, chopped
- 3/4 tsp table salt, divided
- 3 garlic cloves, minced
- 1 tsp minced fresh oregano or 1/4 tsp dried
- 1/4 tsp red pepper flakes

- 1 (28-OZ / 794-g) can whole peeled tomatoes, drained with juice reserved, halved
- 11/2 Ib. (680 g) skinless striped bass, 11/2 inches thick, cut into 2-inch pieces
- 1/4 tsp pepper
- 2 tbsp chopped pitted kalamata olives
- 2 tbsp shredded fresh mint

Direction:

1. For 5 minutes, preheat 1 tsp. of oil in the Instant Pot on the highest sauté setting (or until just smoking). Then add the zucchini and cook for 5 minutes, or until cooked. Remove from heat and put aside.

2. To the now-empty saucepan, add the remaining 1 tbsp of oil, the onion, and 1/4 tsp of salt, and cook on high sauté for approximately 5 minutes, or until the onion is softened. Then, after around 30 seconds, stir in the garlic, oregano, and pepper flakes to release their aroma. Add the tomatoes and their liquid that was saved and stir.

3. Add the remaining 1/2 tsp of salt and pepper to the bass. Bass fillets should be tucked into the tomato sauce, and any extra cooking liquid should be spooned over the fish. Shut the pressure relief valve and secure the lid. Choose zero minutes of cooking time under the high pressure cook setting. When the Instant Pot has achieved pressure, switch it off and quick-release the pressure immediately. Carefully lift the lid and direct the steam away from you.

4. Place bass on a platter, cover with aluminum foil, and let it rest while you prepare the veggies. After adding the zucchini, stir the mixture and let it rest for 5 minutes to cook thoroughly. Add the olives and more salt and pepper to taste, then stir. Toss the

veggies with the remaining oil and serve the bass on top with a sprinkle of mint.

Per Serving

Calories: 302 | fat: 12g | protein: 34g | carbs: 15g | fiber: 6g | sodium: 618mg

Honey-Glazed Chicken Thighs

Prep time: 5 minutes | Cook time: 14 minutes | Serves 4
Ingredients:

- Oil, for spraying
- 4 boneless, skinless chicken thighs, fat trimmed
- 3 tbsp soy sauce
- 1 tbsp balsamic vinegar
- 2 tbsp honey
- 2 tbsp minced garlic
- 1 tsp ground ginger

Direction:

1. The air fryer should be heated to a temperature of at least 400 degrees Fahrenheit (204 degrees Celsius). Prepare the air fryer by lining the basket with parchment paper and spraying it with oil.
2. The chicken should be positioned in the ready-made basket.
3. Prepare as directed, turning after 7 minutes, and cooking for another 7 minutes, or until an instant-read thermometer registers 165 degrees Fahrenheit (74 degrees Celsius) and the juices run clear.
4. For 1–2 minutes over low heat, whisk together the soy sauce, balsamic vinegar, honey, garlic, and ginger in a small saucepan.
5. Just before serving, place the chicken on a serving platter and top with the sauce.

Per Serving
Calories: 286 | fat: 10g | protein: 39g | carbs: 7g | fiber: 0g | sodium: 365mg

Cornish Hens with Honey-Lime Glaze

Prep time: 15 minutes | Cook time: 25 to 30 minutes | Serves 2 to 3

Ingredients:

- 1 Cornish game hen (11/2 to 2 Ib.s / 680 to 907 g)
- 1 tbsp honey
- 1 tbsp lime juice
- 1 tsp poultry seasoning
- Salt and pepper, to taste
- Cooking spray

Direction:

1. Split the chicken in half by cutting through the breast bone and along one side of the spine.
2. Apply the honey-lime juice-poultry seasoning mixture all over the chicken. Add salt and pepper to taste.
3. Coat the inside of the air fryer basket with cooking spray and lay chicken halves skin-side down.
4. Heat an air fryer to 330 degrees Fahrenheit (166 degrees Celsius) and cook for 25 to 30 minutes. When the chicken's fluids flow clean when a fork is inserted into the thigh joint, you know it's ready to eat. Hold off on slicing the hen for at least 5 minutes, preferably 10.

Per Serving

Calories: 287 | fat: 8g | protein: 46g | carbs: 7g | fiber: 0g | sodium: 155mg

Pecan Turkey Cutlets

Prep time: 10 minutes | Cook time: 10 to 12 minutes per batch | Serves 4

Ingredients:

- 3/4 cup of panko bread crumbs
- 1/4 tsp salt
- 1/4 tsp pepper
- 1/4 tsp dry mustard
- 1/4 tsp poultry seasoning
- 1/2 cup of pecans
- 1/4 cup of cornstarch
- 1 egg, beaten
- 1 Ib. (454 g) turkey cutlets, 1/2-inch thick
- Salt and pepper, to taste
- Oil for misting or cooking spray

Direction:

1. Prepare the coating by combining the panko crumbs, 1/4 t salt, 1/4 t pepper, mustard, and poultry spice in a food processor. Crumpets should be finely ground in a food processor. In a food processor, add pecans and pulse briefly until nuts are coarsely chopped. Take it easy and don't force yourself to exhaustion!
2. Set the temperature of the air fryer to 360 degrees Fahrenheit (182 degrees Celsius).
3. Prepare a Cup of cornstarch and another with beaten egg. Put the coating mixture from the food processor onto a third, smaller dish.
4. Salt and pepper the turkey cutlets to your liking.

5. Coat the cutlets with cornstarch, then shake off the extra. Next, coat in beaten egg, and roll in breadcrumbs, pressing to adhere. Put oil or frying spray on both sides and cook them.

6. Cook for 10–12 minutes, or until juices flow clear, using two cutlets per layer in the air fryer basket.

7. To finish cooking the remaining cutlets, repeat procedure 6.

Per Serving

Calories: 340 | fat: 13g | protein: 31g | carbs: 24g | fiber: 4g | sodium: 447mg

Chicken and Vegetable Fajitas

Prep time: 15 minutes | Cook time: 23 minutes | Serves 6
Ingredients:

Chicken:

- 1 Ib. (454 g) boneless, skinless chicken thighs, cut crosswise into thirds
- 1 tbsp vegetable oil
- 41/2 tbsp taco seasoning

Vegetables:

- 1 cup of sliced onion
- 1 cup of sliced bell pepper
- 1 or 2 jalapeños, quartered lengthwise
- 1 tbsp vegetable oil
- 1/2 tsp kosher salt
- 1/2 tsp ground cumin

For Serving:
- Tortillas
- Sour cream
- Shredded cheese

- Guacamole
- Salsa

Direction:

1. To prepare the chicken, combine the chicken, oil, and taco seasoning in a medium Cup and toss to coat.
2. To prepare the veggies, place the onion, bell pepper, jalapeno(s), vegetable oil, salt, and cumin into a separate dish and toss to coat.
3. To use an air fryer, put the chicken in the basket. Air fried at 375 degrees Fahrenheit (191 degrees C) for 10 minutes. Toss the veggies with the spices and oil in the air fryer for a final 13 minutes. Make sure the chicken reaches an internal temperature of 165 degrees Fahrenheit (74 degrees Celsius) by using a meat thermometer.
4. The chicken and veggies should be moved to a serving plate. Wrap in tortillas and top with your preferred fajita ingredients.

Per Serving

Calories: 151 | fat: 8g | protein: 15g | carbs: 4g | fiber: 1g | sodium: 421mg

Coconut Chicken Meatballs

Prep time: 10 minutes | Cook time: 14 minutes | Serves 4
Ingredients:

- 1 Ib. (454 g) ground chicken
- 2 scallions, finely chopped
- 1 cup of chopped fresh cilantro leaves
- 1/4 cup of unsweetened shredded coconut
- 1 tbsp hoisin sauce
- 1 tbsp soy sauce
- 2 tbsp Sriracha or other hot sauce

- 1 tsp toasted sesame oil
- 1/2 tsp kosher salt
- 1 tsp black pepper

Direction:

1. Stir the chicken, scallions, cilantro, coconut, hoisin, soy sauce, Sriracha, sesame oil, salt, and pepper together in a large Cup until well blended (the mixture will be wet and sticky).
2. Line the air fryer's basket with parchment paper. Spoon or use a tsp to put rounded tsp. of the mixture onto the parchment paper.
3. To cook the meatballs in an air fryer, preheat it to 350 degrees Fahrenheit (177 degrees Celsius) for 10 minutes and flip them over halfway through cooking. Cook the meatballs for a further 4 minutes at 400 degrees Fahrenheit (204 degrees Celsius) to brown their exteriors. Use a meat thermometer to confirm the meatballs have achieved an internal temperature of 165ºF (74ºC).
4. Transfer the meatballs to a serving plate. Any residual chicken mixture may be used again.

Per Serving

Calories: 213 | fat: 13g | protein: 21g | carbs: 4g | fiber: 1g | sodium: 501mg

Turkish Chicken Kebabs

Prep time: 30 minutes | Cook time: 15 minutes | Serves 4
Ingredients:

- 1/4 cup of plain Greek yogurt
- 1 tbsp minced garlic
- 1 tbsp tomato paste
- 1 tbsp fresh lemon juice
- 1 tbsp vegetable oil

- 1 tsp kosher salt
- 1 tsp ground cumin
- 1 tsp sweet Hungarian paprika
- 1/2 tsp ground cinnamon
- 1/2 tsp black pepper
- 1/2 tsp cayenne pepper
- 1 Ib. (454 g) boneless, skinless chicken thighs, quartered crosswise

Direction:

1. Yogurt, garlic, tomato paste, lemon juice, vegetable oil, salt, cumin, paprika, cinnamon, black pepper, and cayenne should all be mixed together in a big basin. Mix the spices into the yogurt by stirring.
2. Put the chicken in the Cup and toss it around so it's covered with the marinade. Marinate for 30 minutes at room temperature, or up to 24 hours in the fridge if you cover it.
3. Pile the chicken into the air fryer basket in a single layer. Air fried at 375 degrees Fahrenheit (191 degrees C) for 10 minutes. After 5 minutes, flip the chicken and continue cooking. Make sure the chicken reaches an internal temperature of 165 degrees Fahrenheit (74 degrees Celsius) by using a meat thermometer.

Per Serving
Calories: 188 | fat: 8g | protein: 24g | carbs: 4g | fiber: 1g | sodium: 705mg

Brazilian Tempero Baiano Chicken Drumsticks

Prep time: 30 minutes | Cook time: 20 minutes | Serves 4
Ingredients:

- 1 tsp cumin seeds
- 1 tsp dried oregano

- 1 tsp dried parsley
- 1 tsp ground turmeric
- 1/2 tsp coriander seeds
- 1 tsp kosher salt
- 1/2 tsp black peppercorns
- 1/2 tsp cayenne pepper
- 1/4 cup of fresh lime juice
- 2 tbsp olive oil
- 1-1/2 Ib. (680 g) chicken drumsticks

Direction:

1. Put the cumin, oregano, parsley, turmeric, coriander seeds, salt, pepper, and cayenne into a coffee grinder or spice mill that has been well cleaned. Prepare by grinding until powdery.
2. Mix the ground spices, lime juice, and oil in a small basin. The chicken should be sealed in a plastic bag. Seal the bag and massage the marinade into the chicken until it is evenly distributed. Marinate for 30 minutes at room temperature or up to 24 hours in the fridge.
3. Drumsticks should be cooked with the skin facing up in the air fryer basket. Prepare the chicken legs by frying them in an air fryer at 400 degrees Fahrenheit (204 degrees Celsius) for 20 to 25 minutes before flipping them over. It is recommended to use a meat thermometer to check if the chicken has achieved an internal temperature of 165 degrees Fahrenheit (74 degrees Celsius). Four, have plenty of napkins on hand.

Per Serving

Calories: 267 | fat: 13g | protein: 33g | carbs: 2g | fiber: 1g | sodium: 777mg

Harissa-Rubbed Cornish Game Hens

Prep time: 30 minutes | Cook time: 21 minutes | Serves 4
Ingredients:

Harissa:

- 1/2 cup of olive oil
- 6 cloves garlic, minced
- 2 tbsp smoked paprika
- 1 tbsp ground coriander
- 1 tbsp ground cumin
- 1 tsp ground caraway
- 1 tsp kosher salt
- 1/2 to 1 tsp cayenne pepper

Hens:

- 1/2 cup of yogurt
- 2 Cornish game hens, any giblets removed, split in half lengthwise

Direction:

1. Oil, garlic, paprika, coriander, cumin, caraway, salt, and cayenne are combined in a medium microwave-safe Cup to make harissa. Use a microwave for 1 minute on high, stirring once. You may alternatively heat the oil in a saucepan until it is hot and boiling. Or, if you really can't live without your air fryer, heat the paste in the appliance for 5–6 minutes at 350 °F (177 °C).
2. Put the yogurt and harissa (about 1–2 tsp..) into a small Cup. Mix ingredients together using a whisk. In a plastic bag that can be sealed, toss the chicken halves with the marinade. Keep massaging the bag until all of the pieces are evenly covered with

the coating. Marinate for at least 30 minutes and up to 24 hours at room temperature.

3. In a single layer in the air fryer basket, place the chicken breast halves. (If your air fryer is on the smaller side, you may need to do this in two batches.) Prepare the air fryer for 20 minutes at 400 degrees Fahrenheit (204 degrees Celsius). Check the internal temperature of the game hens using a meat thermometer to make sure they have reached 165 degrees Fahrenheit (74 degrees Celsius).

Per Serving
Calories: 421 | fat: 33g | protein: 26g | carbs: 6g | fiber: 2g | sodium: 683mg

South Indian Pepper Chicken

Prep time: 30 minutes | Cook time: 15 minutes | Serves 4
Ingredients:

Spice Mix:
- 1 dried red Chile, or 1/2 tsp dried red pepper flakes
- 1-inch piece cinnamon or cassia bark
- 11/2 tbsp coriander seeds
- 1 tsp fennel seeds
- 1 tsp cumin seeds
- 1 tsp black peppercorns
- 1/2 tsp cardamom seeds
- 1/4 tsp ground turmeric
- 1 tsp kosher salt

Chicken:

- 1 Ib. (454 g) boneless, skinless chicken thighs, cut crosswise into thirds
- 2 medium onions, cut into 1/2-inch-thick slices

- 1/4 cup of olive oil
- Cauliflower rice, steamed rice, or naan bread, for serving

Direction:

1. To make the spice blend, just combine the dried chili, cinnamon, coriander, fennel, cumin, peppercorns, and cardamom in a tidy coffee or spice grinder. Lightly shake the grinder as you work to ensure that all the seeds and fragments are reaching the blades. Add the salt and turmeric and mix well.

2. In order to marinate the chicken, put the chicken and onions in a plastic bag that can be sealed. Blend in the oil and 1 1/2 tsp. of the spice blend. The chicken should be coated thoroughly after being massaged in a sealed bag. Marinate for 30 minutes at room temperature or up to 24 hours in the fridge.

3. Fill the air fryer basket with the chicken and onions. Air fried at 350 degrees Fahrenheit (177 degrees Celsius) for 10 minutes, stirring once. For 5 minutes, set the oven to 400 degrees Fahrenheit (204 degrees Celsius). Make sure the chicken reaches an internal temperature of 165 degrees Fahrenheit (74 degrees Celsius) by using a meat thermometer.

4. Accompany with your choice of steaming rice, cauliflower rice, or naan.

Per Serving

Calories: 295 | fat: 19g | protein: 24g | carbs: 9g | fiber: 3g | sodium: 694mg

Crispy Dill Chicken Strips

Prep time: 30 minutes | Cook time: 10 minutes | Serves 4
Ingredients:

- 2 whole boneless, skinless chicken breasts (about 1 Ib. / 454 g each), halved lengthwise

- 1 cup of Italian dressing
- 3 cups of finely crushed potato chips
- 1 tbsp dried dill weed
- 1 tbsp garlic powder
- 1 large egg, beaten
- 1 to 2 tbsp oil

Direction:

1. Put the chicken and Italian dressing in a large resealable bag and shake to mix. Put the bag in the fridge for at least an hour to marinate.
2. Put the potato chips, dill, and garlic powder in a shallow Cup and mix well. The beaten egg should be put into a separate, shallow dish.
3. Toss the marinade and dry the chicken. Coat each piece of chicken with egg and then roll it in the potato chip mixture.
4. Start by setting the air fryer temperature to 325 degrees Fahrenheit (163 degrees Celsius). Put parchment paper inside the air fryer basket.
5. Spray oil onto the parchment, then arrange the covered chicken there.
6. Timer for 5 minutes of cooking. After 5 minutes, spray the chicken with oil and flip it over to ensure that all sides are browned and the chicken is no longer pink inside.

Per Serving

Calories: 349 | fat: 16g | protein: 30g | carbs: 20g | fiber: 2g | sodium: 92mg

Simply Terrific Turkey Meatballs

Prep time: 10 minutes | Cook time: 7 to 10 minutes | Serves 4
Ingredients:

- 1 red bell pepper, seeded and coarsely chopped
- 2 cloves garlic, coarsely chopped
- 1/4 cup of chopped fresh parsley
- 11/2 Ib. (680 g) 85% lean ground turkey
- 1 egg, lightly beaten
- 1/2 cup of grated Parmesan cheese
- 1 tsp salt
- 1/2 tsp freshly ground black pepper

Direction:

1. Air fryer temperature should be set at 400 degrees Fahrenheit (204 degrees Celsius).
2. Combine the bell pepper, garlic, and parsley in a food processor with a metal blade. You may finely chop it by pulsing it. Put the veggies in a large basin.
3. Put in the ground turkey, egg, Parmesan, salt, and pepper. Don't rush the process; rather, be slow and thorough. Roll the dough into balls about 11/4 inches in diameter.
4. Spread the meatballs out in a single layer in the air fryer basket, spraying lightly with olive oil spray as needed if working in batches. Air fry for 7 to 10 minutes until lightly browned and a thermometer inserted into the center of a meatball registers 165°F (74°C), stopping halfway through the cooking time to shake the basket.

Per Serving
Calories: 388 | fat: 25g | protein: 34g | carbs: 5g | fiber: 1g | sodium: 527mg

Whole-Roasted Spanish Chicken

Prep time: 1 hour | Cook time: 55 minutes | Serves 4
Ingredients:

- 4 tbsp (1/2 stick) unsalted butter, softened
- 2 tbsp lemon zest
- 2 tbsp smoked paprika
- 2 tbsp garlic, minced
- 1 1/2 tbsp salt
- 1 tsp freshly ground black pepper
- 1 (5-Ib. / 2.3-kg) whole chicken

Direction:

1. Lemon zest, paprika, garlic, salt, and pepper should be added to the butter, which should then be mixed together in a small Cup.
2. Wet a paper towel and pat the chicken dry. Apply the seasoned butter liberally to the chicken using your hands. Place the chicken in the fridge for 30 minutes.
3. Prepare a 425F (220C) oven. Chicken has to be defrosted and let to rest at room temperature for 20 minutes.
4. Cook the chicken for 20 minutes at 400 degrees in a baking dish in the oven. Reduce the heat to 350 degrees Fahrenheit (180 degrees Celsius), and cook the chicken for another 35 minutes.
5. Once the chicken has finished cooking, remove it from the oven and let it rest for 10 minutes before serving.

Per Serving
Calories: 705 | fat: 17g | protein: 126g | carbs: 4g | fiber: 1g | sodium: 880mg

Rosemary Baked Chicken Thighs

Prep time: 20 minutes | Cook time: 20 minutes | Serves 4 to 6
Ingredients:

- 5 tbsp extra-virgin olive oil, divided
- 3 medium shallots, diced
- 4 garlic cloves, peeled and crushed
- 1 rosemary sprig
- 2 to 21/2 Ib. (907 g to 1.1 kg) bone-in, skin-on chicken thighs (about 6 pieces)
- 2 tbsp kosher salt
- 1/4 tsp freshly ground black pepper
- 1 lemon, juiced and zested
- 1/3 cup of low-sodium chicken broth

Direction:

1. Melt 3 tsp. of olive oil in a large skillet or sauté pan over medium heat. Shallots and garlic should be added and cooked for approximately a minute until they release their aroma. Toss in a sprig of rosemary.
2. Sprinkle some salt and pepper on the chicken. Put it on the pan skin-side down and brown it for 3 to 5 minutes.
3. Incorporate lemon juice and zest after the chicken has cooked for half its total time by flipping it over.
4. When the juices run clear, add the chicken stock, cover the pan, and simmer for another 10 to 15 minutes. Serve.

Per Serving
Calories: 294 | fat: 18g | protein: 30g | carbs: 3g | fiber: 1g | sodium: 780mg

Southward Pesto Stuffed Peppers

Prep time: 20 minutes | Cook time: 15 minutes | Serves 4 to 6
Ingredients:

- Nonstick cooking spray
- 3 large bell peppers, halved
- 2 tbsp extra-virgin olive oil, plus more to garnish
- 1/4 cup of cooked chickpeas
- 1/2 shredded carrot
- 2 garlic cloves, minced
- 1 Ib. (454 g) ground turkey or chicken
- Salt
- Freshly ground black pepper
- 1 cup of cooked brown rice
- 1/2 cup of halved cherry tomatoes
- 1/2 zucchini, chopped
- 1 tbsp dried Italian herb medley
- 2 tbsp chopped black olives
- 6 tbsp prepared pesto
- 1/2 cup of shredded Italian cheese blend

Direction:

1. Have ready an oven preheated at 350 degrees Fahrenheit (180 degrees Celsius). Apply a thin layer of cooking spray to a glass baking dish or casserole of similar size.
2. For this, you'll need to boil some water in a medium saucepan and then keep it at a low simmer. Gently submerge the pepper halves in the water using tongs, and cook them for approximately 3 minutes, or until they are just tender enough to be eaten. Take out of the water, and let it drain in a colander.

3. To cook the chickpeas and carrot, heat the olive oil in a large skillet over medium heat. Add the chickpeas and carrot and cook for 5 minutes, or until the vegetables are soft. Sauté the garlic for a minute, or until it becomes aromatic. The turkey should be seasoned with salt and pepper and tossed to ensure uniform cooking.
4. To finish cooking the turkey, add the rice, cherry tomatoes, zucchini, and herbs during the last 5 minutes of cooking.
5. Turn off the heat and mix in the olives. Coat a casserole dish with cooking oil and add the pepper halves you've prepped.
6. The filling should be distributed uniformly among the peppers. Sprinkle some Italian cheese and one tsp. of pesto over the top of each pepper. For 7-10 minutes, depending on how soft you want your peppers, bake them. Wait 10 minutes before serving to let the peppers settle. Add a little of your favorite olive oil and dig in.

Per Serving
Calories: 546 | fat: 38g | protein: 26g | carbs: 28g | fiber: 5g | sodium: 493mg

Bell Pepper and Tomato Chicken

Prep time: 15 minutes | Cook time: 5 hours | Serves 6 to 8
Ingredients:

- 1 medium yellow onion, sliced thickly
- 1 bell pepper, any color, cored, seeded, and sliced thickly
- 4 cloves garlic, minced
- 6 OZs (170 g) pitted black olives, drained
- 1 (28-OZ / 794-g) can stewed tomatoes
- 1 (15-OZ / 425-g) can stewed tomatoes
- 1 (6-OZ / 170-g) can tomato paste

- 1 cup of red or white wine
- 2 tbsp lemon juice
- 4 to 6 boneless, skinless chicken breasts, cut in half
- 1/4 cup of chopped fresh parsley, or 2 tbsp dried parsley
- 1 tbsp dried basil
- 1/2 tsp ground nutmeg
- Sea salt
- Black pepper
- 1 tbsp red pepper flakes

Direction:

1. Put the olives, garlic, onion, and bell pepper in the slow cooker.
2. Put in the canned tomatoes, tomato paste, wine, and fresh lemon juice. Blend ingredients together by stirring.
3. The chicken should be placed into the slow cooker. Use enough liquid to completely coat each item.
4. Parsley, basil, and nutmeg should be sprinkled over top. Add some salt, pepper, and, if you like things spicy, some red pepper flakes. Keep covered and cook for 5 hours on high or 8 hours on low. The chicken has to be cooked all the way through.
5. Spaghetti squash or other cooked pasta are great vehicles for this spicy dish.

Per Serving

Calories: 280 | fat: 7g | protein: 34g | carbs: 15g | fiber: 5g | sodium: 423mg

Garlic Chicken with Couscous

Prep time: 10 minutes | Cook time: 31/2 hours | Serves 4
Ingredients:

- 1 whole chicken, 31/2 to 4 Ib. (1.6 to 1.8 kg), cut into 6 to 8 pieces and patted dry
- Coarse sea salt
- Black pepper
- 1 tbsp extra-virgin olive oil
- 1 medium yellow onion, halved and thinly sliced
- 6 cloves garlic, halved
- 2 tbsp dried thyme
- 1 cup of dry white wine
- 1/3 cup of all-purpose flour
- 1 cup of uncooked couscous
- 1/4 chopped fresh parsley

Direction:

1. Salt and pepper the chicken before cooking.
2. Preheat the oil over medium heat in a big skillet. Chicken should be added skin-side down and cooked in batches for approximately 4 minutes, or until the skin is golden brown. Toss and cook for a another 2 minutes, uncovered.
3. Put the garlic, onion, and thyme in the crock pot.
4. The chicken should be placed skin-side up on top of the slow cooker's ingredients in a single, compact layer. 5. Combine the wine and flour in a small Cup and stir until smooth; then, add to the slow cooker.
5. Cover and simmer for 3 1/2 hours on high or 7 hours on low, or until the chicken is cooked.
6. You should prepare the couscous as directed on the packet.

7. Sprinkle some parsley over the couscous and serve the chicken and sauce on the side.

Per Serving

Calories: 663 | fat: 38g | protein: 46g | carbs: 21g | fiber: 1g | sodium: 166mg

Greek-Style Roast Turkey Breast

Prep time: 10 minutes | Cook time: 71/2 hours | Serves 8
Ingredients:

- 1 (4-Ib. / 1.8-kg) turkey breast, trimmed of fat
- 1/2 cup of chicken stock
- 2 tbsp fresh lemon juice
- 2 cups of chopped onions
- 1/2 cup of pitted kalamata olives
- 1/2 cup of oil-packed sun-dried tomatoes, drained and thinly sliced
- 1 clove garlic, minced
- 1 tsp dried oregano
- 1/2 tsp ground cinnamon
- 1/2 tsp ground dill
- 1/4 tsp ground nutmeg
- 1/4 tsp cayenne pepper
- 1 tsp sea salt
- 1/4 tsp black pepper
- 3 tbsp all-purpose flour

Direction:

1. Get out your slow cooker and toss in the turkey breast, a quarter cup of the chicken stock, the lemon juice, the onions, the Kalamata olives, the garlic, and the sun-dried tomatoes. Add the

spices: oregano, cinnamon, dill, nutmeg, cayenne pepper, salt, and black pepper. Cook, covered, on low heat for 7 hours.

2. In a small basin, mix the remaining 1/4 cup of chicken stock with the flour until a smooth paste forms. Stir the mixture with a whisk until it's uniform. Toss in the slow cooker and stir. Cover and continue cooking for another 30 minutes on low heat.

3. Toss with hot rice, pasta, potatoes, or any other starch of your liking and serve immediately.

Per Serving

Calories: 386 | fat: 7g | protein: 70g | carbs: 8g | fiber: 2g | sodium: 601mg

Chicken Cutlets with Greek Salsa

Prep time: 15 minutes | Cook time: 15 minutes | Serves 2
Ingredients:

- 2 tbsp olive oil, divided
- 1/4 tsp salt, plus additional to taste
- Zest of 1/2 lemon
- Juice of 1/2 lemon
- 8 OZs (227 g) chicken cutlets, or chicken breast sliced through the middle to make 2 thin pieces
- 1 cup of cherry or grape tomatoes, halved or quartered (about 4 OZs / 113 g)
- 1/2 cup of minced red onion (about 1/3 medium onion)
- 1 medium cucumber, peeled, seeded and diced
- 5 to 10 pitted Greek olives, minced (more or less depending on size and your taste)
- 1 tbsp minced fresh parsley
- 1 tbsp minced fresh oregano
- 1 tbsp minced fresh mint

- 1 OZ (28 g) crumbled feta cheese
- 1 tbsp red wine vinegar

Direction:

1. Combine the salt, lemon zest, and lemon juice with 1 tsp. of olive oil in a medium Cup. Put the chicken in the marinade and get to work on the salsa while the chicken cooks.
2. Combine the tomatoes, onion, cucumber, olives, parsley, oregano, mint, feta cheese, and red wine vinegar in a small Cup and toss gently. Rest for at least 30 minutes in the fridge, covered. If more salt or herbs are desired, feel free to add them to the salsa just before serving.
3. In a large nonstick skillet over medium heat, warm the remaining 1 tsp. of olive oil for cooking the chicken. Put in the chicken and cook for three to six minutes per side, depending on how thick the pieces are. It's not time to flip the chicken if it's still sticking to the pan.
4. After the chicken is done cooking, serve it with the salsa on top.

Per Serving
Calories: 357 | fat: 23g | protein: 31g | carbs: 8g | fiber: 2g | sodium: 202mg

Bruschetta Chicken Burgers

Prep time: 15 minutes | Cook time: 15 minutes | Serves 2
Ingredients:

- 1 tbsp olive oil
- 3 tbsp finely minced onion
- 2 garlic cloves, minced
- 1 tsp dried basil
- 1/4 tsp salt
- 3 tbsp minced sun-dried tomatoes packed in olive oil

- 8 OZs (227 g) ground chicken breast
- 3 pieces small mozzarella balls, minced

Direction:

1. Oil the grill grate and preheat the grill to a high temperature (approximately 400oF / 205oC). These may also be cooked in a nonstick skillet if preferred.
2. The olive oil should be heated in a small pan over medium heat. To soften the onion and garlic, add them to the pan and cook for 5 minutes. Insert the basil and mix well. Take it off the stove and put it in a basin.
3. Mix in the dried tomatoes, ground chicken, and salt. Throw in some moss ball chunks.
4. Make two patties from the chicken mixture, each approximately 3/4 of an inch thick.
5. For about five minutes, or until the bottoms are brown, place the burgers on the grill. Grill the burgers for another five minutes, or until an instant-read thermometer registers 165 degrees Fahrenheit (74 degrees Celsius), then flip them over.
6. To cook the patties on the stovetop, heat a nonstick pan over medium heat and add the patties. Get them nice and browned on the bottom by cooking them for 5 to 6 minutes on the first side. The burgers need to achieve an internal temperature of 165 degrees Fahrenheit (74 degrees Celsius), so flip them and cook for another 5 minutes.

Per Serving

Calories: 301 | fat: 17g | protein: 32g | carbs: 6g | fiber: 1g | sodium: 725mg

Skillet Greek Turkey and Rice

Prep time: 20 minutes | Cook time: 30 minutes | Serves 2
Ingredients:

- 1 tbsp olive oil
- 1/2 medium onion, minced
- 2 garlic cloves, minced
- 8 OZs (227 g) ground turkey breast
- 1/2 cup of roasted red peppers, chopped
- 1/4 cup of sun-dried tomatoes, minced
- 1 tsp dried oregano
- 1/2 cup of brown rice
- 1-1/4 cups of low-sodium chicken stock
- Salt
- 2 cups of lightly packed baby spinach

Direction:

1. Olive oil should be heated in a pan over medium heat. Toss in the onion, and cook for 5 minutes. Cook for another 30 seconds after adding the garlic.
2. Once the oil is hot, add the turkey breast and heat for 7 minutes, breaking it up with a spoon to ensure it cooks through.
3. Toss in the roasted red peppers, sun-dried tomatoes, and oregano and mix well. Put in the rice and chicken stock and heat to a boil.
4. Put the lid on the pan and turn the heat down to low. Keep at a low simmer for about 30 minutes, or until the rice is soft. Douse with salt.
5. The spinach should be added to the pan and stirred until it wilts.

Per Serving

Calories: 446 | fat: 17g | protein: 30g | carbs: 49g | fiber: 5g | sodium: 663mg

Salads

Powerhouse Arugula Salad

Prep time: 10 minutes | Cook time: 0 minutes | Serves 4
Ingredients:

- 4 tbsp extra-virgin olive oil
- Zest and juice of 2 clementines or 1 orange (2 to 3 tbsp)
- 1 tbsp red wine vinegar
- 1/2 tsp salt
- 1/4 tsp freshly ground black pepper
- 8 cups of baby arugula
- 1 cup of coarsely chopped walnuts
- 1 cup of crumbled goat cheese
- 1/2 cup of pomegranate seeds

Direction:

1. Olive oil, lemon zest and juice, vinegar, salt, and pepper should be mixed together in a small dish and left away.
2. To serve, toss the arugula, walnuts, goat cheese, and pomegranate seeds together in a large dish. Add the dressing and toss to evenly coat.

Per Serving
Calories: 448 | fat: 41g | protein: 11g | carbs: 13g | fiber: 4g | sodium: 647mg

Tuscan Kale Salad with Anchovies

Prep time: 15 minutes | Cook time: 0 minutes | Serves 4
Ingredients:

- 1 large bunch lacinato or dinosaur kale
- 1/4 cup of toasted pine nuts
- 1 cup of shaved or coarsely shredded fresh Parmesan cheese
- 1/4 cup of extra-virgin olive oil
- 8 anchovy fillets, roughly chopped
- 2 to 3 tbsp freshly squeezed lemon juice
- 2 tbsp red pepper flakes

Direction:

1. Kale leaves should have their tough, central stems removed, and then they should be coarsely torn into 4-by-1-inch strips. Mix the kale, pine nuts, and cheese in a large Cup.
2. Olive oil, anchovies, lemon juice, and red pepper flakes are combined in a small basin and whisked together (if using). Pour over salad and toss to evenly distribute. Allow to remain at room temperature for 30 minutes before serving, then toss one more before dishing out.

Per Serving
Calories: 333 | fat: 27g | protein: 16g | carbs: 12g | fiber: 4g | sodium: 676mg

Traditional Greek Salad

Prep time: 10 minutes | Cook time: 0 minutes | Serves 4
Ingredients:

- 2 large English cucumbers
- 4 Roma tomatoes, quartered
- 1 green bell pepper, cut into 1- to 1-1/2-inch chunks
- 1/4 small red onion, thinly sliced
- 4 OZs (113 g) pitted Kalamata olives
- 1/4 cup of extra-virgin olive oil
- 2 tbsp freshly squeezed lemon juice
- 1 tbsp red wine vinegar
- 1 tbsp chopped fresh oregano or 1 tsp dried oregano
- 1/4 tsp freshly ground black pepper
- 4 OZs (113 g) crumbled traditional feta cheese

Direction:

1. The cucumbers should be halved lengthwise and then sliced into half-moons about an inch thick. Make room in a big dish.
2. Toss in the chopped olives, red onion, bell pepper, and tomato quarters.
3. Olive oil, lemon juice, vinegar, oregano, and black pepper should be combined in a small basin and whisked together. Spread it over the veggies and toss to coat.
4. To serve, divide the salad into plates and sprinkle each with 28 grams of feta.

Per Serving
Calories: 256 | fat: 22g | protein: 6g | carbs: 11g | fiber: 3g | sodium: 476mg

Orange-Tarragon Chicken Salad Wrap

Prep time: 15 minutes | Cook time: 0 minutes | Serves 4
Ingredients:

- 1/2 cup of plain whole-milk Greek yogurt
- 2 tbsp Dijon mustard
- 2 tbsp extra-virgin olive oil
- 2 tbsp chopped fresh tarragon or 1 tsp dried tarragon
- 1/2 tsp salt
- 1/4 tsp freshly ground black pepper
- 2 cups of cooked shredded chicken
- 1/2 cup of slivered almonds
- 4 to 8 large Bibb lettuce leaves, tough stem removed
- 2 small ripe avocados, peeled and thinly sliced
- Zest of 1 clementine, or 1/2 small orange

Direction:

1. Whisk together the yogurt, mustard, olive oil, tarragon, orange zest, salt, and pepper in a medium Cup until smooth and creamy.
2. Then, toss in the shredded chicken and the almonds and mix to combine.
3. To make the wraps, divide the chicken salad mixture among the lettuce leaves, and then top with the avocado slices.

Per Serving
Calories: 491 | fat: 38g | protein: 28g | carbs: 14g | fiber: 9g | sodium: 454mg

Israeli Salad with Nuts and Seeds

Prep time: 15 minutes | Cook time: 0 minutes | Serves 4
Ingredients:

- 1/4 cup of pine nuts
- 1/4 cup of shelled pistachios
- 1/4 cup of coarsely chopped walnuts
- 1/4 cup of shelled pumpkin seeds
- 1/4 cup of shelled sunflower seeds
- 2 large English cucumbers, unpeeled and finely chopped
- 1 pint cherry tomatoes, finely chopped
- 1/2 small red onion, finely chopped
- 1/2 cup of finely chopped fresh flat-leaf Italian parsley
- 1/4 cup of extra-virgin olive oil
- 2 to 3 tbsp freshly squeezed lemon juice
- 1 tsp salt
- 1/4 tsp freshly ground black pepper
- 4 cups of baby arugula

Direction:

1. Toast the pine nuts, pistachios, walnuts, pumpkin seeds, and sunflower seeds in a large dry pan over medium heat until brown and aromatic, 5 to 6 minutes. Take away from the stove, then.
2. Combine the cucumber, tomato, red onion, and parsley in a large Cup.
3. Olive oil, lemon juice, salt, and pepper may be mixed together in a small Cup. Mix it up with the chopped veggies.
4. Toss in the arugula and any toasted nuts or seeds, and mix everything well. Eat warm or cold.

Per Serving

Calories: 404 | fat: 36g | protein: 10g | carbs: 16g | fiber: 5g | sodium: 601mg

Pistachio-Parmesan Kale-Arugula Salad

Prep time: 20 minutes |Cook time: 0 minutes| Serves: 6
Ingredients:

- 6 cups of raw kale, center ribs removed and discarded, leaves coarsely chopped
- 1/4 cup of extra-virgin olive oil
- 2 tbsp freshly squeezed lemon juice
- 1/2 tsp smoked paprika
- 2 cups of arugula
- 1/3 cup of unsalted shelled pistachios
- 6 tbsp grated Parmesan or Pecorino Romano cheese

Direction:

1. Mix the kale, oil, lemon juice, and smoked paprika in a large salad Cup. For around 15 seconds, knead the leaves with your hands to ensure that they are fully covered. You should wait 10 minutes before preparing the greens.
2. Add the arugula and pistachios just before serving and toss gently. A tsp. of grated cheese should be sprinkled over each plate of salad before it is served.

Per Serving
Calories: 150 | fat: 14g | protein: 4g | carbs: 5g | fiber: 1g | sodium: 99mg

Melon Caprese Salad

Prep time: 20 minutes |Cook time: 0 minutes| Serves: 6
Ingredients:

- 1 cantaloupe, quartered and seeded
- 1/2 small seedless watermelon
- 1 cup of grape tomatoes
- 2 cups of fresh mozzarella balls (about 8 OZs / 227 g)
- 1/3 cup of fresh basil or mint leaves, torn into small pieces
- 2 tbsp extra-virgin olive oil
- 1 tbsp balsamic vinegar
- 1/4 tsp freshly ground black pepper
- 1/4 tsp kosher or sea salt

Direction:

1. Make cantaloupe balls by scooping them out with a melon baller or a metal tsp-sized measuring spoon. A single cantaloupe should provide 2.5–3 cups of purée. (Instead of rolling the melon into balls, you may instead chop it into smaller pieces.) Place them in a big colander set over a big basin for serving.
2. Use the same technique to ball up or slice the watermelon into bite-sized pieces; you should have enough for around 2 cups. Combine the cantaloupe cubes and watermelon balls in the colander.
3. Just wait 10 minutes for the fruit to drain. The juice may be stored in the fridge and used later in smoothies or other drinks. After drying it off, place the chopped fruit inside.
4. To the fruit Cup, put the tomatoes, mozzarella, basil, oil, vinegar, pepper, and salt. Stir gently until combined, then serve.

Per Serving

Calories: 297 | fat: 12g | protein: 14g | carbs: 39g | fiber: 3g | sodium: 123mg

Chopped Greek Antipasto Salad

Prep time: 20 minutes |Cook time: 0 minutes| Serves: 6
Ingredients:

For the Salad:
- 1 head Bibb lettuce or 1/2 head romaine lettuce, chopped
- 1/4 cup of loosely packed chopped basil leaves
- 1 (15-OZ / 425-g) can chickpeas, drained and rinsed
- 1 (14-OZ / 397-g) can artichoke hearts, drained and halved
- 1pint grape tomatoes, halved
- 1 seedless cucumber, peeled and chopped
- 1/2 cup of cubed feta cheese
- 1 (21/4-OZ / 35-g) can sliced black olives

For the Dressing:
- 3 tbsp extra-virgin olive oil
- 1 tbsp red wine vinegar
- 1 tbsp freshly squeezed lemon juice
- 1 tbsp chopped fresh oregano or 1/2 tsp dried oregano
- 1 tsp honey
- 1/4 tsp freshly ground black pepper

Direction:

1. Mix the basil and lettuce in a medium basin. Disperse on a hulking plate or a massive salad dish. Over the lettuce, make little heaps of the chickpeas, artichoke hearts, tomatoes, cucumber, feta, and olives.

2. Mix the oil, vinegar, lemon juice, oregano, honey, and pepper in a small pitcher or dish. Serve with the salad or drizzle over the salad just before serving.

Per Serving

Calories: 267 | fat: 13g | protein: 11g | carbs: 31g | fiber: 11g | sodium: 417mg

Mediterranean Potato Salad

Prep time: 10 minutes |Cook time: 20 minutes| Serves: 6
Ingredients:

- 2 Ib. (907 g) Yukon Gold baby potatoes, cut into 1-inch cubes
- 3 tbsp freshly squeezed lemon juice
- 3 tbsp extra-virgin olive oil
- 1 tbsp olive brine
- 1/4 tsp kosher or sea salt
- 1 (21/4-OZ / 35-g) can sliced olives
- 1 cup of sliced celery (about 2 stalks) or fennel
- 2 tbsp chopped fresh oregano
- 2 tbsp torn fresh mint

Direction:

1. Place potatoes in a medium saucepan and fill with cold water until it reaches a level that's about an inch over the potatoes. Turn the heat up high to bring the potatoes to a boil, then reduce to a simmer. Cook at a low boil for 12–15 minutes, or until the potatoes are soft enough to be easily pierced with a fork.
2. While the potatoes are in the oven, make the dressing by combining the lemon juice, oil, olive brine, and salt in a small dish. Next, place the potatoes in a colander to drain, and then transfer them to a serving dish. Quickly drizzle the dressing, approximately 3 tsp. worth, over the potatoes. Olives and celery

should be folded in gently. Fourth, just before serving, carefully fold in the oregano, mint, and the remaining dressing.

Per Serving

Calories: 192 | fat: 8g | protein: 3g | carbs: 28g | fiber: 4g | sodium: 195mg

Roasted Broccoli Panzanella Salad

Prep time: 10 minutes |Cook time: 20 minutes| Serves: 4
Ingredients:

- 1 Ib. (454 g) broccoli (about 3 medium stalks), trimmed, cut into 1-inch florets and 1/2-inch stem slices
- 3 tbsp extra-virgin olive oil, divided
- 1 pint cherry or grape tomatoes
- 1-1/2 tbsp honey, divided
- 3 cups of cubed whole-grain crusty bread
- 1 tbsp balsamic vinegar
- 1/2 tsp freshly ground black pepper
- 1/4 tsp kosher or sea salt
- Grated Parmesan cheese (or other hard cheese) and chopped fresh oregano leaves, for serving

Direction:

1. Put a large, high-sided baking sheet in the oven. Put the pan in the oven and preheat it to 450 degrees Fahrenheit (235 degrees Celsius).
2. Sprinkle 1 tbsp. of the oil over the broccoli and toss it in a large Cup. Coat toss.
3. Carefully take out the heated baking sheet and transfer the broccoli onto it using a slotted spoon, reserving some of the oil in the Cup. Put the tomatoes in the same Cup as the rest of the ingredients, and toss to coat with the remaining oil (do not add

any more oil). Spread the broccoli out on a baking pan and toss the tomatoes with 1 tsp of honey.

4. Stir halfway through cooking time, and roast for 15 minutes. Take out the baking sheet and fill it with cubed bread. Roast for a further 3 minutes. When the broccoli has browned at the tips and is tender-crisp when pierced with a fork, it is done.

5. Put the veggie medley in a big, flat dish or on a serving platter.

6. Mix the vinegar, the remaining 1/2 tsp honey, the pepper, and salt with the remaining 2 tbsp of oil in a small basin. Drizzle it over the salad and gently mix it in. Serve with a sprinkle of cheese and some oregano, if you want..

Per Serving

Calories: 197 | fat: 12g | protein: 7g | carbs: 19g | fiber: 5g | sodium: 296mg

Easy Greek Salad

Prep time: 10 minutes | Cook time: 0 minutes | Serves 4 to 6
Ingredients:

- 1 head iceberg lettuce
- 1 pint (2 cups of) cherry tomatoes
- 1 large cucumber
- 1 medium onion
- 1/2 cup of extra-virgin olive oil
- 1/4 cup of lemon juice
- 1 tsp salt
- 1 clove garlic, minced
- 1 cup of Kalamata olives, pitted
- 1 (6-OZ / 170-g) package feta cheese, crumbled

Direction:

1. Put the lettuce in a big salad dish and chop it into 1-inch pieces.

2. Tomatoes, after halved, may be added to a salad.
3. Cucumbers should be cut into small pieces and added to the salad as a garnish.
4. Toss the onion into the salad as thin slices.
5. Mix the olive oil, lemon juice, salt, and garlic together in a separate small Cup. Toss the salad lightly after pouring the dressing over it to get a uniform coating. 6. Kalamata olives and feta cheese provide a delicious finishing touch to the salad.

Per Serving
Calories: 297 | fat: 27g | protein: 6g | carbs: 11g | fiber: 3g | sodium: 661mg

Citrusy Spinach Salad

Prep time: 10 minutes | Cook time: 5 minutes | Serves 4
Ingredients:

- 1 large ripe tomato
- 1 medium red onion
- 1/2 tsp fresh lemon zest
- 3 tbsp balsamic vinegar
- 1/4 cup of extra-virgin olive oil
- 1/2 tsp salt
- 1 Ib. (454 g) baby spinach, washed, stems removed

Direction:

1. Slice the onion thinly and slice the tomato into little bite-sized pieces.
2. Mix the lemon zest, balsamic vinegar, olive oil, and salt in a small Cup.
3. In a large Cup, combine the spinach, tomato, and onion. Toss the salad gently to coat with the dressing, then serve.

Per Serving

Calories: 172 | fat: 14g | protein: 4g | carbs: 10g | fiber: 4g | sodium: 389mg

Classic Tabouli

Prep time: 30 minutes | Cook time: 0 minutes | Serves 8 to 10
Ingredients:

- 1 cup of bulgur wheat, grind
- 4 cups of Italian parsley, finely chopped
- 2 cups of ripe tomato, finely diced
- 1 cup of green onion, finely chopped
- 1/2 cup of lemon juice
- 1/2 cup of extra-virgin olive oil
- 1 1/2 tbsp salt
- 1 tsp dried mint

Direction:

1. Start with placing the bulgur in a small Cup before you start chopping the veggies. Drain and let sit in the basin under cold running water while you prepare the rest of the ingredients.
2. Combine the bulgur, parsley, tomatoes, and green onion in a big Cup.
3. Mix the lemon juice, olive oil, salt, and mint in a small Cup.
4. After combining the tomatoes, onions, and bulgur, pour the dressing over the salad and toss to coat. To taste, add more salt. Serve right away, or refrigerate for up to 2 days.

Per Serving
Calories: 207 | fat: 14g | protein: 4g | carbs: 20g | fiber: 5g | sodium: 462mg

Mediterranean Quinoa and Garbanzo Salad

Prep time: 10 minutes | Cook time: 30 minutes | Serves 8
Ingredients:

- 4 cups of water
- 2 cups of red or yellow quinoa
- 2 tbsp salt, divided
- 1 cup of thinly sliced onions
- 1 (16-OZ / 454-g) can garbanzo beans, rinsed and drained
- 1/3 cup of extra-virgin olive oil
- 1/4 cup of lemon juice
- 1 tsp freshly ground black pepper

Direction:

1. Bring the water to a boil in a 3-quart saucepan set over medium heat.
2. Stir in the quinoa and 1 t of salt. To cook on low heat for 15–20 minutes, stir, then cover.
3. Immediately remove the quinoa from the heat, fluff it with a fork, cover it back up, and let it sit for 5-10 minutes.
4. Prepare a big Cup for mixing the quinoa, onions, and chickpeas.
5. Combine the olive oil, lemon juice, remaining 1 t of salt, and the black pepper in a separate small Cup and whisk to combine.
6. Once you've added the dressing, toss the quinoa mixture lightly. Prepare hot or cold.

Per Serving
Calories: 318 | fat: 13g | protein: 9g | carbs: 43g | fiber: 6g | sodium: 585mg

Yellow and White Hearts of Palm Salad

Prep time: 10 minutes | Cook time: 0 minutes | Serves 4
Ingredients:

- 2 (14-OZ / 397-g) cans hearts of palm, drained and cut into 1/2-inch-thick slices
- 1 avocado, cut into 1/2-inch pieces
- 1 cup of halved yellow cherry tomatoes
- 1/2 small shallot, thinly sliced
- 1/4 cup of coarsely chopped flat-leaf parsley
- 2 tbsp low-fat mayonnaise
- 2 tbsp extra-virgin olive oil
- 1/4 tsp salt
- 1/8 tsp freshly ground black pepper

Direction:

1. Mix the hearts of palm, avocado, tomatoes, shallot, and parsley in a big Cup. Mayonnaise, olive oil, salt, and pepper should be whisked together in a smaller Cup before being added to the larger Cup.

Per Serving
Calories: 192 | fat: 15g | protein: 5g | carbs: 14g | fiber: 7g | sodium: 841mg

Spanish Potato Salad

Prep time: 10 minutes | Cook time: 10 minutes | Serves 6 to 8
Ingredients:

- 4 russet potatoes, peeled and chopped
- 3 large hard-boiled eggs, chopped
- 1 cup of frozen mixed vegetables, thawed
- 1/2 cup of plain, unsweetened, full-fat Greek yogurt
- 5 tbsp pitted Spanish olives
- 1/2 tsp freshly ground black pepper
- 1/2 tsp dried mustard seed
- 1/2 tbsp freshly squeezed lemon juice
- 1/2 tsp dried dill
- Salt
- Freshly ground black pepper

Direction:

2. Potatoes should be boiled for 5–7 minutes, until they are just fork-tender. Overcooking them would be a bad idea.
3. While the potatoes are in the oven, combine the other ingredients (eggs, veggies, yogurt, olives, pepper, mustard, lemon juice, and dill) in a big dish. Use salt and pepper to taste. Add the potatoes to the big Cup after they have cooled down a little, stir, and serve.

Per Serving
Calories: 192 | fat: 5g | protein: 9g | carbs: 30g | fiber: 2g | sodium: 59mg

No-Mayo Florence Tuna Salad

Prep time: 10 minutes | Cook time: 0 minutes | Serves 4
Ingredients:

4 cups of spring mix greens

1 (15-OZ / 425-g) can cannellini beans, drained

2 (5-OZ / 142-g) cans water-packed, white albacore tuna, drained

2/3 cup of crumbled feta cheese

1/2 cup of thinly sliced sun-dried tomatoes

1/4 cup of sliced pitted kalamata olives

1/4 cup of thinly sliced scallions, both green and white parts

3 tbsp extra-virgin olive oil

1/2 tsp dried cilantro

2 or 3 leaves thinly chopped fresh sweet basil

1 lime, zested and juiced

Kosher salt

Freshly ground black pepper

Direction:

1. Greens, beans, tuna, feta, tomatoes, olives, scallions, olive oil, cilantro, basil, lime juice, and lime zest are mixed together in a large Cup. Sprinkle some salt and pepper on it, stir it up, and dig in!

Per Serving 1 cup of:
Calories: 355 | fat: 19g | protein: 22g | carbs: 25g | fiber: 8g | sodium: 744mg

Tricolor Tomato Summer Salad

Prep time: 10 minutes | Cook time: 0 minutes | Serves 3 to 4
Ingredients:

- 1/4 cup of while balsamic vinegar
- 2 tbsp Dijon mustard
- 1 tbsp sugar
- 1/2 tsp freshly ground black pepper
- 1/2 tsp garlic salt
- 1/4 cup of extra-virgin olive oil
- 11/2 cups of chopped orange, yellow, and red tomatoes
- 1/2 cucumber, peeled and diced
- 1 small red onion, thinly sliced
- 1/4 cup of crumbled feta

Direction:

2. Mix together the vinegar, mustard, sugar, pepper, and garlic salt in a small Cup. Then, gradually add the olive oil while stirring.
3. Tomatoes, cucumbers, and red onion should be combined in a big dish. Douse the salad with the dressing. Add the feta cheese crumbles (if using) and toss again before serving.

Per Serving
Calories: 246 | fat: 18g | protein: 1g | carbs: 19g | fiber: 2g | sodium: 483mg

Tomato and Pepper Salad

Prep time: 10 minutes | Cook time: 0 minutes | Serves 6
Ingredients:

- 3 large yellow peppers
- 1/4 cup of olive oil
- 1 small bunch fresh basil leaves
- 2 cloves garlic, minced
- 4 large tomatoes, seeded and diced
- Sea salt and freshly ground pepper, to taste

Direction:

1. Turn on your broiler's high heat and broil the peppers until they are blackened on all sides.
2. Take off the stove and place in a paper bag. Keep peppers sealed and chilled. Once the peppers have cooled, remove the stems and seeds before chopping them.
3. Combine half of the peppers with the olive oil, basil, and garlic in a food processor and pulse several times to make a dressing.
4. Toss the remaining peppers with the tomatoes and the dressing. Add some freshly ground pepper and sea salt to the salad. Let the salad sit out at room temperature for a while before serving.

Per Serving
Calories: 129 | fat: 9g | protein: 2g | carbs: 11g | fiber: 2g | sodium: 8mg

Warm Fennel, Cherry Tomato, and Spinach Salad

Prep time: 15 minutes | Cook time: 0 minutes | Serves 2
Ingredients:

- 4 tbsp chicken broth
- 4 cups of baby spinach leaves
- 10 cherry tomatoes, halved
- Sea salt and freshly ground pepper, to taste
- 1 fennel bulb, sliced
- 1/4 cup of olive oil
- Juice of 2 lemons

Direction:

1. Chicken stock should be heated over medium heat in a large sauté pan. The tomatoes and spinach can be cooked together until the spinach is wilted. Use a generous amount of fine sea salt and freshly ground pepper.
2. Take the spinach and tomatoes from the heat and mix them with the sliced fennel. Warm the fennel in the pan before transferring to a large serving basin.
3. Serve immediately with a drizzle of olive oil and a squeeze of lemon.

Per Serving
Calories: 319 | fat: 28g | protein: 5g | carbs: 18g | fiber: 6g | sodium: 123mg

Cinnamon-Apple Chips

Prep time: 10 minutes | Cook time: 32 minutes | Serves 4
Ingredients:

- Oil, for spraying
- 2 Red Delicious or Honeycrisp apples
- 1/4 tsp ground cinnamon, divided

Direction:

1. Prepare the air fryer by spraying the basket with oil and lining it with parchment paper.
2. Cut off the apples' ragged ends. Cut the apples into extremely thin slices using a mandolin set to its thinnest setting or a sharp knife. Throw away the centers. Spread half the apple slices in a single layer in the prepared basket and sprinkle with half the cinnamon.
3. To prevent the apples from rolling about the kitchen as they cook, place a metal air fryer trivet on top of them.
4. Cook in an air fryer at 300 degrees Fahrenheit (149 degrees Celsius) for 16 minutes, turning once after 8 minutes. Replace the cinnamon and apple slices with the rest.
5. Serve after it has cooled to room temperature. As the chips cool, they will harden.

Per Serving
Calories: 63 | fat: 0g | protein: 0g | carbs: 15g | fiber: 3g | sodium: 1mg

Sea Salt Potato Chips

Prep time: 30 minutes | Cook time: 27 minutes | Serves 4
Ingredients:

- Oil, for spraying
- 4 medium yellow potatoes
- 1 tbsp oil
- 1/8 to 1/4 tsp fine sea salt

Direction:

1. Spray oil sparingly into the air fryer basket and line it with parchment paper.
2. Slice the potatoes extremely thinly using a mandolin or a very sharp knife.
3. Put the slices into the basin of cold water and let them sit there for around 20 minutes.
4. The potatoes should be drained, then moved to a dish covered with paper towels and dried off well.
5. After salting the potatoes, drizzle them with oil and toss them to coat. Move to the waiting basket.
6. Cook in an air fryer for 20 minutes at 200 degrees Fahrenheit (93 degrees Celsius). Toss the chips and raise the temperature to 400 degrees Fahrenheit (204 degrees Celsius) for another 5 to 7 minutes, until they reach the desired crispiness.

Per Serving
Calories: 194 | fat: 4g | protein: 4g | carbs: 37g | fiber: 5g | sodium: 90mg

Taco-Spiced Chickpeas

Prep time: 5 minutes | Cook time: 17 minutes | Serves 3
Ingredients:

- Oil, for spraying
- 1 (151/2-OZ / 439-g) can chickpeas, drained
- 1 tsp chili powder
- 1/2 tsp ground cumin
- 1/2 tsp salt
- 1/2 tsp granulated garlic
- 2 tbsp lime juice

Direction:

1. Spray oil sparingly into the air fryer basket and line it with parchment paper. Put the chickpeas in the hamper you have just set up.
2. Shake or mix the chickpeas and spritz gently with oil every 5 to 7 minutes throughout the air-frying process, which takes 17 minutes at 390oF (199oC).
3. Combine the spices (chili powder, cumin, salt, and garlic) in a small Cup.
4. Sprinkle half of the spice combination over the chickpeas with 2 to 3 minutes left on the cooking timer. Put away the food.
5. Put the chickpeas in a medium Cup and add the remaining seasoning blend and the lime juice. Serve at once.

Per Serving
Calories: 208 | fat: 4g | protein: 11g | carbs: 34g | fiber: 10g | sodium: 725mg

Ranch Oyster Snack Crackers

Prep time: 3 minutes | Cook time: 12 minutes | Serves 6
Ingredients:

- Oil, for spraying
- 1/4 cup of olive oil
- 2 tbsp dry ranch seasoning
- 1 tsp chili powder
- 1/2 tsp dried dill
- 1/2 tsp granulated garlic
- 1/2 tsp salt
- 1 (9-OZ / 255-g) bag oyster crackers

Direction:

1. Make sure the air fryer is at 325 degrees Fahrenheit (163 degrees Celsius). Spray oil sparingly into the air fryer basket and line it with parchment paper.
2. Using a large Cup, combine the olive oil, ranch seasoning, chili powder, dill, garlic, and salt. Put in the crackers and mix until they are all covered.
3. Put the ingredients in the basket.
4. Shake or stir every three to four minutes for ten to twelve minutes until crisp and golden brown.

Per Serving
Calories: 261 | fat: 13g | protein: 4g | carbs: 32g | fiber: 1g | sodium: 621mg

Garlic-Parmesan Croutons

Prep time: 3 minutes | Cook time: 12 minutes | Serves 4
Ingredients:

- Oil, for spraying
- 4 cups of cubed French bread
- 1 tbsp grated Parmesan cheese
- 3 tbsp olive oil
- 1 tbsp granulated garlic
- 1/2 tsp unsalted salt

Direction:

1. Spray oil sparingly into the air fryer basket and line it with parchment paper.
2. Toss the bread cubes, Parmesan cheese, olive oil, garlic, and salt together with your hands in a large basin until all ingredients are uniformly coated. Place the bread cubes that have been coated into the basket.
3. Crisp and golden-brown results may be achieved by air frying at 350°F (177°C) for 10–12 minutes while stirring once after 5 minutes.

Per Serving
Calories: 220 | fat: 12g | protein: 5g | carbs: 23g | fiber: 1g | sodium: 285mg

Parmesan French Fries

Prep time: 10 minutes | Cook time: 25 minutes | Serves 2 to 3
Ingredients:

- 2 to 3 large russet potatoes, peeled and cut into 1/2-inch sticks
- 2 tbsp vegetable or canola oil
- 3/4 cup of grated Parmesan cheese
- 1/2 tsp salt
- Freshly ground black pepper, to taste
- 1 tsp fresh chopped parsley

Direction:

1. While you are peeling and chopping the potatoes, have a big kettle of salted water boiling on the stove. While the air fryer is heating up to temperature (about 400F/204C), blanch the potatoes in the boiling salted water for 4 minutes. The potatoes should be drained and then rinsed in cold water. Use a fresh dish towel to thoroughly dry them.
2. Oil the dry potato sticks well and set them in the air fryer basket. Shake the basket a few times throughout the air-frying process to ensure that the fries brown evenly.
3. Mix the grated Parmesan, salt, and pepper together. Put the fries in the air fryer and cook for 2 minutes. At this point, sprinkle the Parmesan cheese mixture over the fries. Air fried for a further 2 minutes, until the cheese has melted and just begins to brown, then toss the fries to cover them evenly with the cheese mixture. When the fries are done, sprinkle them with chopped parsley and serve with more grated Parmesan cheese if desired.

Per Serving
Calories: 252 | fat: 11g | protein: 13g | carbs: 27g | fiber: 2g | sodium: 411mg

Lemon-Pepper Chicken Drumsticks

Prep time: 30 minutes | Cook time: 30 minutes | Serves 2
Ingredients:

- 2 tbsp freshly ground coarse black pepper
- 1 tsp baking powder
- 1/2 tsp garlic powder
- 4 chicken drumsticks
- Kosher salt, to taste
- 1 lemon

Direction:

1. Mix the baking powder, garlic powder, and pepper in a small basin. Arrange the drumsticks in a single layer on a dish, then use tongs to flip each one in the baking powder mixture until it is equally coated. You should refrigerate the drumsticks for at least an hour and up to a whole night.
2. Season the drumsticks with salt and place them in the air fryer, bone side up, resting against the side of the air fryer basket. Air fried at 375 °F (191 °C) for 30 minutes, or until well cooked and the outside is crisp.
3. While the drumsticks are still hot, place them on a serving plate and sprinkle the lemon zest over them. Drumsticks should be served hot, with lemon cut into wedges.

Per Serving
Calories: 438 | fat: 24g | protein: 48g | carbs: 6g | fiber: 2g | sodium: 279mg

Garlic Edamame

Prep time: 5 minutes | Cook time: 10 minutes | Serves 4
Ingredients:

- Olive oil
- 1 (16-OZ / 454-g) bag frozen edamame in pods
- 1/2 tsp salt
- 1/2 tsp garlic salt
- 1/4 tsp freshly ground black pepper
- 1/2 tsp red pepper flakes

Direction:

1. Lightly coat the basket of the air fryer with olive oil spray.
2. Spray some olive oil into a medium Cup and add the frozen edamame. Coat toss.
3. Combine the salt, garlic salt, black pepper, and red pepper flakes in a separate small Cup (if using). Toss the edamame with the sauce until it is well covered.
4. Spread out half of the edamame in the air fryer basket. Don't put too much in the basket.
5. Crisp in the oven at 375 degrees Fahrenheit (191 degrees Celsius) for 5 minutes. Cook for a further 3–5 minutes, shaking the basket occasionally, or until the edamame begins to brown and become crispy.
6. You may then immediately serve the rest of the edamame after a second round of cooking.

Per Serving
Calories: 125 | fat: 5g | protein: 12g | carbs: 10g | fiber: 5g | sodium: 443mg

Black Bean Corn Dip

Prep time: 10 minutes | Cook time: 10 minutes | Serves 4
Ingredients:

- 1/2 (15-OZ / 425-g) can black beans, drained and rinsed
- 1/2 (15-OZ / 425-g) can corn, drained and rinsed
- 1/4 cup of chunky salsa
- 2 OZs (57 g) reduced-fat cream cheese, softened
- 1/4 cup of shredded reduced-fat Cheddar cheese
- 1/2 tsp ground cumin
- 1/2 tsp paprika
- Salt and freshly ground black pepper, to taste

Direction:

1. Make sure the air fryer is at 325 degrees Fahrenheit (163 degrees Celsius).
2. Combine the black beans, corn, salsa, cream cheese, Cheddar cheese, cumin, and paprika in a medium Cup and stir to combine. Add the salt and pepper and whisk to incorporate.
3. Mix everything together and place in a baking dish.
4. Heat for about 10 minutes in an air fryer after placing baking dish in its basket.
5. Assemble while still hot.

Per Serving
Calories: 119 | fat: 2g | protein: 8g | carbs: 19g | fiber: 6g | sodium: 469mg

Crunchy Tex-Mex Tortilla Chips

Prep time: 5 minutes | Cook time: 5 minutes | Serves 4
Ingredients:

- Olive oil
- 1/2 tsp salt
- 1/2 tsp ground cumin
- 1/2 tsp chili powder
- 1/2 tsp paprika
- Pinch cayenne pepper
- 8 (6-inch) corn tortillas, each cut into 6 wedges

Direction:

1. Prepare the frying basket with a quick spray of olive oil.
2. Combine the salt, cumin, chili powder, paprika, and cayenne pepper in a small Cup.
3. To use an air fryer, put down a single layer of tortilla wedges in the basket. Oil the tortillas gently and sprinkle with the spice blend. To prevent the tortillas from burning, cook them in batches.
4. Cook in an air fryer for 2–3 minutes at 375°F (191°C). After 2–3 minutes, give the basket a shake and continue cooking until the chips are a golden brown and crispy. Keep a watchful eye on them to prevent them from burning.

Per Serving
Calories: 118 | fat: 1g | protein: 3g | carbs: 25g | fiber: 3g | sodium: 307mg

Mexican Potato Skins

Prep time: 10 minutes | Cook time: 55 minutes | Serves 6
Ingredients:

- Olive oil
- 6 medium russet potatoes, scrubbed
- Salt and freshly ground black pepper, to taste
- 1 cup of fat-free refried black beans
- 1 tbsp taco seasoning
- 1/2 cup of salsa
- 3/4 cup of reduced-fat shredded Cheddar cheese

Direction:

1. Olive oil the air fryer basket gently.
2. Oil and season potatoes. Fork-pierce each potato.
3. Air-fry the potatoes. Air fried at 400oF (204oC) until fork-tender, 30–40 minutes. Potato size determines cooking time. The air fryer gives potatoes a crispier skin than the microwave or oven.
4. Mix beans and taco spice in a small dish while the potatoes cook. Leave potatoes to cool.
5. Half each potato lengthwise. To keep the potato skins intact, scoop off most of the insides, leaving 1/4 inch.
6. Salt and black pepper the potato skins. Oil the potato skins. Batch-cook them.
7. Air fried them skin-side down for 8–10 minutes.
8. On a work surface, spoon 1/2 tbsp of seasoned refried black beans into each skin. Top each with 2 tbsp salsa and 1 tbsp grated Cheddar.
9. Layer loaded potato skins in the air fryer. Mist oil. 10. Air fried until the cheese melts and bubbles, 2–3 minutes.

Per Serving

Calories: 239 | fat: 2g | protein: 10g | carbs: 46g | fiber: 5g | sodium: 492mg

Greens Chips with Curried Yogurt Sauce

Prep time: 10 minutes | Cook time: 5 to 6 minutes | Serves 4
Ingredients:

- 1 cup of low-fat Greek yogurt
- 1 tbsp freshly squeezed lemon juice
- 1 tbsp curry powder
- 1/2 bunch curly kale, stemmed, ribs removed and discarded, leaves cut into 2- to 3-inch pieces
- 1/2 bunch chard, stemmed, ribs removed and discarded, leaves cut into 2- to 3-inch pieces
- 1-1/2 tbsp olive oil

Direction:

1. In a small Cup, whisk together the yogurt, lemon juice, and curry powder. Set aside.
2. In a large Cup, mix the kale and chard with the olive oil, massaging the oil into the leaves with your hands. This softens leaf chips by breaking up fibers.
3. Air fried the greens in batches at 390oF (199oC) for 5–6 minutes until crisp, stirring the basket once. Yogurt sauce.

Per Serving

Calories: 98 | fat: 4g | protein: 7g | carbs: 13g | fiber: 4g | sodium: 186mg

Vegetable Pot Stickers

Prep time: 12 minutes | Cook time: 11 to 18 minutes | Makes 12 pot stickers

Ingredients:

1. 1 cup of shredded red cabbage
2. 1/4 cup of chopped button mushrooms
3. 1/4 cup of grated carrot
4. 2 tbsp minced onion
5. 2 garlic cloves, minced
6. 2 tbsp grated fresh ginger
7. 12 gyoza/pot sticker wrappers
8. 2-1/2 tbsp olive oil, divided

Direction:

1. In a baking pan, mix the red cabbage, mushrooms, carrot, onion, garlic, and ginger. Add 1 tbsp of water. Air fried at 370oF (188oC) until crisp-tender. Drain.
2. Place each pot sticker wrapper on a work surface. Top each wrapper with a scant 1 tbsp of the filling. Fold half of the wrapper over the other side to make a half circle. Wet one edge and push both together.
3. 11/4 tbsp olive oil to another pan. Put half of the pot stickers, seam-side up, in the pan. Air fried for 5 minutes, or until the bottoms are light golden brown. Add 1 tbsp of water and return the pan to the air fryer.
4. Air fry for 4–6 minutes until hot. Repeat with the remaining pot stickers, remaining 1-1/4 tbsp of oil, and another tbsp of water. Serve now.

Per Serving (1 pot stickers)
Calories: 36 | fat: 1g | protein: 1g | carbs: 6g | fiber: 0g | sodium: 49mg

Roasted Mushrooms with Garlic

Prep time: 3 minutes | Cook time: 22 to 27 minutes | Serves 4
Ingredients:

- 16 garlic cloves, peeled
- 2 tbsp olive oil, divided
- 16 button mushrooms
- 1/2 tsp dried marjoram
- 1/8 tsp freshly ground black pepper
- 1 tbsp white wine or low-sodium vegetable broth

Direction:

1. In a baking pan, mix garlic with 1 tsp olive oil. Air fry at 350oF (177oC) for 12 minutes.
2. Mushrooms, marjoram, and pepper. Coat. Drizzle with white wine and the remaining 1 tsp olive oil.
3. Roast for 10–15 minutes more in the air fryer until the mushrooms and garlic cloves are tender. Serve.

Per Serving
Calories: 57 | fat: 3g | protein: 3g | carbs: 7g | fiber: 1g | sodium: 6mg

Marinated Feta and Artichokes

Prep time: 10 minutes | Cook time: 0 minutes | Makes 11/2 cups of
Ingredients:

- 4 OZs (113 g) traditional Greek feta, cut into 1/2-inch cubes
- 4 OZs (113 g) drained artichoke hearts, quartered lengthwise
- 1/3 cup of extra-virgin olive oil
- Zest and juice of 1 lemon
- 2 tbsp roughly chopped fresh rosemary
- 2 tbsp roughly chopped fresh parsley

- 1/2 tsp black peppercorns

Direction:

1. Mix feta and artichoke hearts in a glass Cup. Toss the feta gently with olive oil, lemon zest and juice, rosemary, parsley, and peppercorns.
2. Refrigerate for 4–4 days. Remove from fridge 30 minutes before serving.

Per Serving

Calories: 108 | fat: 9g | protein: 3g | carbs: 4g | fiber: 1g | sodium: 294mg

Tuna Croquettes

Prep time: 40 minutes | Cook time: 25 minutes | Makes 36 croquettes

Ingredients:

- 6 tbsp extra-virgin olive oil, plus 1 to 2 cups of
- 5 tbsp almond flour, plus 1 cup of, divided
- 1-1/4 cups of heavy cream
- 1 (4-OZ / 113-g) can olive oil-packed yellowfin tuna
- 1 tbsp chopped red onion
- 2 tbsp minced capers
- 1/2 tsp dried dill
- 1/4 tsp freshly ground black pepper
- 2 large eggs
- 1 cup of panko breadcrumbs

Direction:

1. Heat 6 tbsp olive oil in a large skillet on medium-low. Add 5 tbsp almond flour and simmer, stirring regularly, until a smooth paste forms and the flour browns slightly, 2–3 minutes.

2. Increase the heat to medium-high and slowly add the heavy cream, whisking until smooth and thickened, 4 to 5 minutes.

3. Add tuna, red onion, capers, dill, and pepper after removing from heat. 4. Pour the mixture into an olive oil-coated 8-inch square baking dish and cool to room temperature. Cover and chill for 4–24 hours.

4. Prepare three Cups for croquettes. Beat eggs. Add the remaining almond flour to another. Third, add panko. Parchment a baking sheet.

5. Spoon approximately a tsp. of chilled prepared dough into the flour mixture and roll to coat. Shake excess and form an oval with your hands.

6. Dip the croquette in egg and panko. Repeat with remaining dough on prepared baking sheet.

7. Heat 1 to 2 cups of olive oil to approximately 1 inch deep in a small saucepan over medium-high heat. Smaller pans use less oil, but more each batch.

8. Throw a pinch of panko into saucepan to test oil readiness. Fry in oil that sizzles. Sinking indicates unreadiness. Fry 3 or 4 croquettes at a time, depending on pan size, till golden brown. To avoid burning, adjust oil temperature periodically. Reduce the heat if the croquettes brown rapidly.

Per Serving
Calories: 271 | fat: 26g | protein: 5g | carbs: 6g | fiber: 1g | sodium: 89mg

Citrus-Marinated Olives

**Prep time: 10 minutes | Cook time: 0 minutes | Makes 2 cups of
Ingredients:**

- 2 cups of mixed green olives with pits
- 1/4 cup of red wine vinegar
- 1/4 cup of extra-virgin olive oil
- 4 garlic cloves, finely minced
- Zest and juice of 2 clementines or 1 large orange
- 1 tsp red pepper flakes
- 2 bay leaves
- 1/2 tsp ground cumin
- 1/2 tsp ground allspice

Direction:

1. In a large glass Cup or jar, add the olives, vinegar, oil, garlic, orange zest and juice, red pepper flakes, bay leaves, cumin, and allspice and stir well. Cover and refrigerate for at least 4 hours or up to a week to enable the olives to marinade, stirring again before serving.

Per Serving (1/4 cup of)
Calories: 112 | fat: 10g | protein: 1g | carbs: 5g | fiber: 2g | sodium: 248mg

Manchego Crackers

Prep time: 15 minutes | Cook time: 15 minutes | Makes 40 crackers

Ingredients:

- 4 tbsp butter, at room temperature
- 1 cup of finely shredded Manchego cheese
- 1 cup of almond flour
- 1 tsp salt, divided
- 1/4 tsp freshly ground black pepper
- 1 large egg

Direction:

2. Mix butter and shredded cheese with an electric mixer until smooth.
3. Almond flour, 1/2 tsp salt, and pepper in a small basin. Mix the cheese and almond flour mixture until it forms a ball.
4. Roll into an 11/2-inch-thick cylinder on parchment or plastic wrap. Refrigerate for 1 hour.
5. Preheat oven to 350oF (180oC). Line two baking sheets with parchment or silicone mats.
6. Whisk the egg and 1/2 tsp salt in a separate dish to produce the egg wash. 6. Cut 1/4-inch-thick circles of chilled dough and put on prepared baking pans.
7. Egg wash the crackers and bake till golden and crispy, 12–15 minutes. Remove from oven and cool on wire rack.
8. Serve warm or refrigerate for up to a week.

Per Serving

Calories: 73 | fat: 7g | protein: 3g | carbs: 1g | fiber: 1g | sodium: 154mg

Burrata Caprese Stack

Prep time: 5 minutes | Cook time: 0 minutes | Serves 4
Ingredients:

- 1 large organic tomato, preferably heirloom
- 1/2 tsp salt
- 1/4 tsp freshly ground black pepper
- 1 (4-OZ / 113-g) ball burrata cheese
- 8 fresh basil leaves, thinly sliced
- 2 tbsp extra-virgin olive oil
- 1 tbsp red wine or balsamic vinegar

Direction:

1. Salt and pepper four thick slices of tomato, eliminating the tough central core. Serve the tomatoes seasoned-side up.
2. Slice the burrata into four thick slices and arrange one on each tomato slice on a separate rimmed platter. Top each with one-quarter of the basil and any remaining burrata cream from the rimmed plate.
3. Serve with olive oil and vinegar

Per Serving
Calories: 109 | fat: 7g | protein: 9g | carbs: 3g | fiber: 1g | sodium: 504mg

Salmon-Stuffed Cucumbers

Prep time: 10 minutes | Cook time: 0 minutes | Serves 4
Ingredients:

- 2 large cucumbers, peeled
- 1 (4-OZ / 113-g) can red salmon
- 1 medium very ripe avocado, peeled, pitted, and mashed

- 1 tbsp extra-virgin olive oil
- Zest and juice of 1 lime
- 3 tbsp chopped fresh cilantro
- 1/2 tsp salt
- 1/4 tsp freshly ground black pepper

Direction:

1. Slice the cucumber into 1-inch segments and scoop the seeds out of the core with a spoon. Stand them up on a platter.
2. Mix salmon, avocado, olive oil, lime zest and juice, cilantro, salt, and pepper in a medium Cup until smooth. 3. Serve cooled cucumber slices with salmon mixture in the middle.

Per Serving

Calories: 173 | fat: 13g | protein: 8g | carbs: 8g | fiber: 4g | sodium: 420mg

Goat Cheese–Mackerel Pâté

Prep time: 10 minutes | Cook time: 0 minutes | Serves 4
Ingredients:

- 4 OZs (113 g) olive oil-packed wild-caught mackerel
- 2 OZs (57 g) goat cheese
- Zest and juice of 1 lemon
- 2 tbsp chopped fresh parsley
- 2 tbsp chopped fresh arugula
- 1 tbsp extra-virgin olive oil
- 2 tbsp chopped capers
- 1 to 2 tbsp fresh horseradish
- Crackers, cucumber rounds, endive spears, or celery, for serving

Direction:

1. Combine mackerel, goat cheese, lemon zest and juice, parsley, arugula, olive oil, capers, and horseradish in a food processor, blender, or large basin with immersion blender (if using). Blend till creamy.
2. Crackers, cucumber rounds, endive spears, or celery.
3. Refrigerate covered for 1 week.

Per Serving

Calories: 142 | fat: 10g | protein: 11g | carbs: 1g | fiber: 0g | sodium: 203mg

Taste of the Mediterranean Fat Bombs

Prep time: 15 minutes | Cook time: 0 minutes | Makes 6 fat bombs
Ingredients:

- 1 cup of crumbled goat cheese
- 4 tbsp jarred pesto
- 12 pitted Kalamata olives, finely chopped
- 1/2 cup of finely chopped walnuts
- 1 tbsp chopped fresh rosemary

Direction:

1. Mix goat cheese, pesto, and olives in a medium Cup with a fork. Harden in the fridge for 4 hours.
2. Shape the mixture into six 3/4-inch balls with your hands. The mixture will stick.
3. In a small Cup, mix walnuts and rosemary and coat goat cheese balls.
4. Store fat bombs in the fridge for a week or in the freezer for a month.

Per Serving

Calories: 235 | fat: 22g | protein: 10g | carbs: 2g | fiber: 1g | sodium: 365mg

Lemony Garlic Hummus

Prep time: 5 minutes |Cook time: 0 minutes| Serves: 6
Ingredients:

- 1 (15-OZ / 425-g) can chickpeas, drained, liquid reserved
- 3 tbsp freshly squeezed lemon juice
- 2 tbsp peanut butter
- 3 tbsp extra-virgin olive oil, divided
- 2 garlic cloves
- 1/4 tsp kosher or sea salt Raw veggies or whole-grain crackers, for serving

Direction:

1. Combine the chickpeas, lemon juice, peanut butter, oil, and garlic in a food processor. 1 minute. Rubber spatula the Cup's sides. Process another minute until smooth.
2. Place in a Cup, drizzle with the remaining 1 tbsp olive oil, sprinkle with salt, and serve with crackers or vegetables.

Per Serving
Calories: 192 | fat: 11g | protein: 6g | carbs: 18g | fiber: 5g | sodium: 258mg

Honey-Rosemary Almonds

Prep time: 5 minutes |Cook time: 10 minutes| Serves: 6
Ingredients:

- 1 cup of raw, whole, shelled almonds
- 1 tbsp minced fresh rosemary
- 1/4 tsp kosher or sea salt

- 1 tbsp honey
- Nonstick cooking spray

Direction:

1. Almonds, rosemary, and salt in a large pan over medium heat. Stir regularly for 1 minute.
2. Drizzle in the honey and heat for another 3 to 4 minutes, stirring regularly, until the almonds are covered and just beginning to color around the edges.
3. Stop cooking. Spread almonds on a nonstick pan using a spatula. 10 minutes to cool. Serve almonds broken.
4. Serving

Per Serving

Calories: 149 | fat: 12g | protein: 5g | carbs: 8g | fiber: 3g | sodium: 97mg

Fig-Pecan Energy Bites

Prep time: 20 minutes |Cook time: 0 minutes| Serves: 6
Ingredients:

- 3/4 cup of diced dried figs
- 1/2 cup of chopped pecans
- 1/4 cup of rolled oats
- 2 tbsp ground flaxseed or wheat germ
- 2 tbsp powdered or regular peanut butter
- 2 tbsp honey

Direction:

1. Mix figs, pecans, oats, flaxseed, and peanut butter in a medium Cup. Add honey and blend. Press figs and nuts into honey and powdered ingredients with a wooden spoon. 2. Divide the dough equally into four basin portions. Don't overwent your hands or

the dough may stick. Roll three energy bites from each of the four dough portions using your hands.

2. Serve immediately or freeze for 5 minutes to firm the bits. Bites may be refrigerated for one week in a sealed container.

Per Serving

Calories: 196 | fat: 10g | protein: 4g | carbs: 26g | fiber: 4g | sodium: 13mg

Crunchy Orange-Thyme Chickpeas

Prep time: 5 minutes |Cook time: 20 minutes| Serves: 4
Ingredients:

- 1 (15-OZ / 425-g) can chickpeas, drained and rinsed
- 2 tbsp extra-virgin olive oil
- 1/4 tsp dried thyme or 1/2 tsp chopped fresh thyme leaves
- 1/8 tsp kosher or sea salt
- Zest of 1/2 orange

Direction:

1. Turn the oven temperature up to 450F (235C).
2. Lay the chickpeas out on a clean dish towel and gently wipe them until they are dry.
3. Prepare a big, rimmed baking sheet for the chickpeas. Drizzle with oil and season with thyme and salt. Zest half of the orange over the chickpeas using a Microplate or citrus zester. Use your hands to get a good blend.
4. After 10 minutes, remove the pan from the oven and shake it gently while wearing an oven mitt. (Leave the sheet in the oven.) Add another 10 minutes to the baking time. (Careful!) try some of the chickpeas. If you want them extra crunchy, bake them for 3 minutes after they get brown.

Per Serving

Calories: 167 | fat: 5g | protein: 7g | carbs: 24g | fiber: 7g | sodium: 303mg

Creamy Traditional Hummus

Prep time: 5 minutes | Cook time: 0 minutes | Serves 8
Ingredients:

- 1 (15-OZ / 425-g) can garbanzo beans, rinsed and drained
- 2 cloves garlic, peeled
- 1/4 cup of lemon juice
- 1 tsp salt
- 1/4 cup of plain Greek yogurt
- 1/2 cup of tahini paste
- 2 tbsp extra-virgin olive oil, divided

Direction:

1. Add garbanzo beans, garlic cloves, lemon juice, and salt to a food processor with a chopping blade. Blend until smooth.
2. Scrape processor sides. Blend Greek yogurt, tahini paste, and 1 tbsp olive oil for another minute until smooth.
3. Serve hummus. Add the remaining olive oil.

Per Serving
Calories: 189 | fat: 13g | protein: 7g | carbs: 14g | fiber: 4g | sodium: 313mg

Smoky Baba Ghanoush

Prep time: 50 minutes | Cook time: 40 minutes | Serves 6
Ingredients:

- 2 large eggplants, washed
- 1/4 cup of lemon juice
- 1 tsp garlic, minced
- 1 tsp salt
- 1/2 cup of tahini paste
- 3 tbsp extra-virgin olive oil

Direction:

1. Grill entire eggplants over low heat on a gas cooktop or grill. Turn the eggplant after 5 minutes to fry evenly. Repeat for 40 minutes.
2. Place eggplants on a dish or Cup and cover with plastic wrap. Wait 5–10 minutes.
3. Peel and discard the eggplants' scorched skin with your fingers. Cut the stem.
4. Chop eggplants in a food processor. Pulse lemon juice, garlic, salt, and tahini paste 5–7 times.
5. Serve eggplant combination. Drizzle olive oil. Serve cold.

Per Serving
Calories: 230 | fat: 18g | protein: 5g | carbs: 16g | fiber: 7g | sodium: 416mg

Lemony Olives and Feta Medley

Prep time: 10 minutes | Cook time: 0 minutes | Serves 8
Ingredients:

- 1 (1-Ib. / 454-g) block of Greek feta cheese
- 3 cups of mixed olives, drained from brine; pitted preferred
- 1/4 cup of extra-virgin olive oil
- 3 tbsp lemon juice
- 1 tsp grated lemon zest
- 1 tsp dried oregano
- Pita bread, for serving

Direction:

1. Put 1/2-inch feta cheese cubes in a large basin.
2. Set aside feta with olives.
3. Mix olive oil, lemon juice, lemon zest, and oregano in a small Cup.
4. Toss the feta cheese and olives in the dressing.
5. Serve flat bread.

Per Serving
Calories: 269 | fat: 24g | protein: 9g | carbs: 6g | fiber: 2g | sodium: 891mg

Quick Garlic Mushrooms

Prep time: 10 minutes | Cook time: 10 minutes | Serves 4 to 6
Ingredients:

- 2 Ib. (907 g) cremini mushrooms, cleaned
- 3 tbsp unsalted butter
- 2 tbsp garlic, minced
- 1/2 tsp salt

- 1/2 tsp freshly ground black pepper

Direction:

1. Put each mushroom half in a basin, stem to top.
2. Medium-heat a big sauté pan.
3. Stirring periodically, cook butter and garlic for 2 minutes.
4. Toss mushrooms, salt, and garlic butter in the pan. 7–8 minutes, stirring every 2 minutes.
5. Pour mushrooms into a serving dish. pepper.

Per Serving

Calories: 183 | fat: 9g | protein: 9g | carbs: 10g | fiber: 3g | sodium: 334mg

Seared Halloumi with Pesto and Tomato

Prep time: 2 minutes | Cook time: 5 minutes | Serves 2
Ingredients:

- 3 OZs (85 g) Halloumi cheese, cut crosswise into 2 thinner, rectangular pieces
- 2 tbsp prepared pesto sauce, plus additional for drizzling if desired
- 1 medium tomato, sliced

Direction:

1. Put the Halloumi slices in a nonstick pan that's been heated over medium heat. After 2 minutes, examine the cheese to see whether the bottom has become golden. If the underside is golden, turn the slices, top with 1 tsp of pesto, and fry for another 2 minutes.
2. Tomato slices and a dollop of pesto, if using, can be served on the side.

Per Serving

Calories: 177 | fat: 14g | protein: 10g | carbs: 4g | fiber: 1g | sodium: 233mg

Arabic-Style Spiced Roasted Chickpeas

Prep time: 15 minutes | Cook time: 35 minutes | Serves 2
For the Seasoning Mix:
Ingredients:

- 3/4 tsp cumin
- 1/2 tsp coriander
- 1/2 tsp salt
- 1/4 tsp freshly ground black pepper
- 1/4 tsp paprika
- 1/4 tsp cardamom
- 1/4 tsp cinnamon
- 1/4 tsp allspice

For the Chickpeas:
- 1 (15-OZ / 425-g) can chickpeas, drained and rinsed
- 1 tbsp olive oil
- 1/4 tsp salt

Direction:

Make the Seasoning Mix:

1. Mix the paprika, cardamom, cinnamon, cloves, and allspice with the paprika, coriander, salt, freshly ground black pepper, and cumin in a small Cup. Combine everything by stirring it together well, then putting it aside.

Make the Chickpeas

2. Preheat the oven to 400oF (205oC) with the rack in the center. Line a baking sheet with parchment.

3. To dry the washed chickpeas, pat them with paper towels or roll them in a clean kitchen towel.

4. Season the chickpeas with olive oil and salt in a dish.

5. Roast the chickpeas for 25–35 minutes on the prepared baking sheet, turning them once or twice. Most should be light brown. Taste one or two to make sure they're crisp.

6. Sprinkle the spice mix on the roasted chickpeas. Lightly mix. Taste and add salt if required. Hot.

Per Serving
Calories: 268 | fat: 11g | protein: 11g | carbs: 35g | fiber: 10g | sodium: 301mg

Apple Chips with Chocolate Tahini

Prep time: 10 minutes | Cook time: 0 minutes | Serves 2
Ingredients:

- 2 tbsp tahini
- 1 tbsp maple syrup
- 1 tbsp unsweetened cocoa powder
- 1 to 2 tbsp warm water 2 medium apples
- 1 tbsp roasted, salted sunflower seeds

Direction:

1. Mix tahini, maple syrup, and cocoa powder in a small Cup. Slowly add warm water until it drizzles. Microwaving won't thin it.

2. To produce chips, cut the apples crosswise into circular slices and then in half.

3. Pour chocolate tahini sauce over apple chips on a dish.

4. Sunflower seeds with apple crisps.

Per Serving

Calories: 261 | fat: 11g | protein: 5g | carbs: 43g | fiber: 8g | sodium: 21mg

Herbed Labneh Vegetable Parfaits

Prep time: 15 minutes | Cook time: 0 minutes | Serves 2
Ingredients:

For the Labneh:
- 8 OZs (227 g) plain Greek yogurt
- Generous pinch salt
- 1 tsp za'atar seasoning
- 1 tsp freshly squeezed lemon juice
- Pinch lemon zest

For the Parfaits:
- 1/2 cup of peeled, chopped cucumber
- 1/2 cup of grated carrots
- 1/2 cup of cherry tomatoes, halved

Direction:

Make the Labneh:

1. Insert cheesecloth into a sieve and set it over a basin.
2. Greek yogurt and salt should be mixed together and strained through cheesecloth. Put it in a sealed container and chill for a full day.
3. When you're ready, remove the labneh from its packaging and transfer it to a Cup. The za'atar, lemon juice, and lemon zest should all be combined and stirred together.
4. Preparing the Parfaits First, split the cucumber into two transparent glasses.
5. Put three tsp.. of labneh on top of each serving of cucumber.
6. Put a carrot in each of the glasses.

7. Spread another 3 tsp.. of the labneh on top.

8. Cherry tomatoes are the perfect finishing touch for your parfaits.

Per Serving

Calories: 143 | fat: 7g | protein: 5g | carbs: 16g | fiber: 2g | sodium: 187mg

Heart-Healthful Trail Mix

Prep time: 15 minutes | Cook time: 30 minutes | Serves 10
Ingredients:

- 1 cup of raw almonds
- 1 cup of walnut halves
- 1 cup of pumpkin seeds
- 1 cup of dried apricots, cut into thin strips
- 1 cup of dried cherries, roughly chopped
- 1 cup of golden raisins
- 2 tbsp extra-virgin olive oil
- 1 tsp salt

Direction:

1. The oven has to be preheated to 300F (150C). Arrange aluminum foil on a baking pan. Second, mix the apricots, cherries, almonds, walnuts, pumpkin seeds, and raisins in a big Cup. Toss everything together with clean hands after adding the olive oil. Toss in the salt and stir to disperse.

2. Spread the nut mixture out in a single layer on the baking sheet and bake for approximately 30 minutes, or until the fruits start to turn golden. Reserve the baking sheet at room temperature while cooling. Put away in a big, sealable plastic bag or airtight container.

Per Serving

Calories: 346 | fat: 20g | protein: 8g | carbs: 39g | fiber: 5g | sodium: 240mg

Marinated Olives and Mushrooms

Prep time: 10 minutes | Cook time: 0 minutes | Serves 8
Ingredients:

- 1 Ib. (454 g) white button mushrooms
- 1 Ib. (454 g) mixed, high-quality olives
- 2 tbsp fresh thyme leaves
- 1 tbsp white wine vinegar
- 1/2 tbsp crushed fennel seeds
- Pinch chili flakes
- Olive oil, to cover
- Sea salt and freshly ground pepper, to taste

Direction:

1. Mushrooms need to be cleaned in cold water and then patted dry.
2. Place everything in a glass jar or other airtight container. Sprinkle with salt and freshly ground pepper and cover with olive oil. In order to mix the components, give it a good shake. Marinate for at least an hour before serving. Prepare at ambient temperature.

Per Serving
Calories: 61 | fat: 4g | protein: 2g | carbs: 5g | fiber: 2g | sodium: 420mg

Warm Olives with Rosemary and Garlic

Prep time: 5 minutes | Cook time: 3 minutes | Serves 4
Ingredients:

- 1 tbsp olive oil
- 1 clove garlic, chopped
- 2 sprigs fresh rosemary
- 1/4 tsp salt
- 1 cup of whole cured black olives, such as Kalamata

Direction:

1. Olive oil, in a medium saucepan, should be heated over moderate heat. Mix in the salt, garlic, and rosemary. Turn the heat down low and cook for 1 minute while stirring constantly.
2. Put in the olives and heat them for about 2 minutes, stirring occasionally.
3. Using a slotted spoon, transfer the olives from the pan to a serving Cup. Warm up some olives and serve them with the rosemary and garlic.

Per Serving
Calories: 71 | fat: 7g | protein: 1g | carbs: 3g | fiber: 1g | sodium: 441mg

Croatian Red Pepper Dip

Prep time: 10 minutes | Cook time: 30 minutes | Serves 4 to 6
Ingredients:

- 4 or 5 medium red bell peppers
- 1 medium eggplant
- 1/4 cup of olive oil, divided
- 1 tsp salt, divided
- 1/2 tsp freshly ground black pepper, divided
- 4 cloves garlic, minced
- 1 tbsp white vinegar

Direction:

1. High-temperature broiler.
2. Foil a large baking sheet.
3. 2 tbsp olive oil, 1/2 tsp salt, and 1/4 tsp pepper on the peppers and eggplant. Broil the peppers and eggplant, flipping every few minutes, until the skins are browned. Peppers take 10 minutes, eggplant 20.
4. After the peppers are properly roasted, take them from the baking pan, put them in a dish, cover with plastic wrap, and steam while the eggplant cooks. Remove the eggplant from the oven when it is totally roasted and tender.
5. Peel the peppers' charred skins when they're cold. Discard burned skins. Food processor the pepper seeds.
6. Pulse the garlic in the food processor to roughly chop the veggies. Process the remaining olive oil, vinegar, and 1/2 tsp salt to a smooth purée.
7. Simmer the vegetable mixture in a medium saucepan over medium-high heat. Simmer on medium-low for 30 minutes, stirring periodically. Cool from heat. Serve room-temperature.

Per Serving

Calories: 144 | fat: 11g | protein: 2g | carbs: 12g | fiber: 5g | sodium: 471mg

Charred Eggplant Dip with Feta and Mint

Prep time: 5 minutes | Cook time: 20 minutes | Makes about 11/2 cups of
Ingredients:

- 1 medium eggplant
- 2 tbsp lemon juice
- 1/4 cup of olive oil
- 1/2 cup of crumbled feta cheese
- 1/2 cup of finely diced red onion
- 3 tbsp chopped fresh mint leaves
- 1 tbsp finely chopped flat-leaf parsley
- 1/4 tsp cayenne pepper
- 3/4 tsp salt

Direction:

1. High-temperature broiler.
2. Foil a baking sheet.
3. Poke the eggplant several times with a fork on the prepared baking sheet. Cook under the broiler, turning about every 5 minutes, until the eggplant is charred on all sides and very soft in the center, about 15 to 20 minutes total. Remove from the oven and put aside until cool enough to handle.
4. After the eggplant cools, split it in half lengthwise and scoop out the meat, discarding the scorched peel.
5. Fork-mash the lemon juice and olive oil into a rough purée. Add the cheese, onion, mint, parsley, cayenne, and salt. 6. Serve at room temperature.

Per Serving 1/2 cup of:

Calories: 71 | fat: 6g | protein: 2g | carbs: 3g | fiber: 2g | sodium: 237mg

Spanish-Style Pan-Roasted Cod

Prep time: 15 minutes | Cook time: 25 minutes | Serves 4
Ingredients:

- 4 tbsp olive oil
- 8 garlic cloves, minced
- 1/2 small onion, finely chopped
- 1/2 Ib. (227 g) small red or new potatoes, quartered
- 1 (141/2-OZ / 411-g) can low-sodium diced tomatoes, with their juices
- 16 pimiento-stuffed low-salt Spanish olives, sliced
- 4 tbsp finely chopped fresh parsley
- 4 (4-OZ / 113-g) cod fillets, about 1 inch thick
- Salt and freshly ground black pepper

Direction:

1. In a 10-inch skillet, heat 2 tbsp olive oil and garlic over medium heat. Cook for 1–2 minutes, taking care not to burn the garlic.
2. On medium-high heat, add the onion, potatoes, tomatoes with their juices, olives, and 3 tbsp parsley. Start boiling. Reduce the heat to a simmer, cover, and cook for 15–18 minutes until the potatoes are cooked. Transfer the skillet mixture to a large Cup and keep heated. Clean the skillet and put it back on the burner.
3. Over medium-high heat, heat the skillet's remaining 2 tbsp olive oil. Add the fish to the pan and season with salt and pepper. After 2–3 minutes, turn the fish and cook for 2–3 more minutes until it flakes easily.
4. Top each dish with a fish fillet and tomato mixture. Serve with 1 tbsp parsley.

Per Serving 1 cup of:
Calories: 297 | fat: 20g | protein: 9g | carbs: 20g | fiber: 4g | sodium: 557mg

Salmon Niçoise Salad with Dijon-Chive Dressing

Prep time: 10 minutes | Cook time: 20 minutes | Serves 4
Ingredients:

- 1 Ib. (454 g) baby or fingerling potatoes
- 1/2 Ib. (227 g) green beans
- 6 tbsp olive oil
- 4 (4-OZ / 113-g) salmon fillets
- 1/4 tsp freshly ground black pepper
- 2 tbsp Dijon mustard
- 3 tbsp red wine vinegar
- 1 tbsp, plus 1 tsp finely chopped fresh chives
- 1 head romaine lettuce, sliced cross-wise
- 2 hard-boiled eggs, quartered
- 1/4 cup of Niçoise or other small black olives
- 1 cup of cherry tomatoes, quartered

Direction:

1. The potatoes should be placed in a big saucepan and covered with cold water. Cook for 12-15 minutes, or until soft when poked with a fork, after the water has been brought to a boil and then reduced to a simmer. Wait until it is cold enough to handle, then drain and cut it into cubes. Putting aside.
2. In the meanwhile, get the water boiling in a medium saucepan. Green beans should be added and cooked for three minutes. It may be stopped from cooking by draining and rinsing with cold water. Don't bother with right now.

3. One tsp. of the olive oil should be heated over medium heat in a large pan. Pepper the fish before cooking. After preheating the pan, place the salmon fillets skin-side down and cook for 4–5 minutes on each side. The food should be transferred to a dish and kept warm.

4. Mix the mustard, vinegar, 1 tsp. of the chives, and the remaining 5 tsp.. of olive oil in a small dish.

5. Cut the lettuce in half and place it on four separate dishes. Put a fillet of salmon on each person's plate. To serve, toss the potatoes, green beans, eggs, olives, and tomatoes with the dressing and divide among plates.

6. When ready to serve, sprinkle with the remaining 1 t of chives.

Per Serving 1 cup of:

Calories: 398 | fat: 25g | protein: 15g | carbs: 30g | fiber: 8g | sodium: 173mg

Conclusion

Consistent weight loss is a challenge. It's important to find a weight-loss plan that works for you but doesn't add too much stress to your life. There is a wide variety of options available, and although many of them may be effective, others may be too challenging or even harmful to your health.

This guide will examine the Weight Watchers program and the incredible benefits it may provide to your health. While some diet regimens may limit what you may eat, this one does not. Treats like those are OK to have on occasion, but only if you exercise moderation.

This guide will explain the ins and outs of the Weight Watchers program, including how to track your progress, earn and spend points, and build a healthy diet and eating plan into your daily routine. As a result, adopting a healthy lifestyle may aid in weight loss, energy levels, and other areas of improvement.

If you've been on a never-ending hunt for a diet plan that will help you lose weight and is also easy to stick to, Weight Watchers may be the solution you've been looking for all along. Learn all you need to know about weight loss, maintaining a healthy lifestyle, and having more fun in life with this comprehensive guide.

I really hope you enjoyed this book and that you took away some helpful information from it. If you could, I'd really value a review of this book. The purchase of this book is much appreciated.